Preparing for Pregnancy

A Health Primer for Parents-to-be

Professor Geoffrey Chamberlain

with a foreword by Sir George Pinker, KCVO

FONTANA/Collins

First published in 1990 by Fontana Paperbacks
8 Grafton Street, London W1X 3LA

Copyright © Geoffrey Chamberlain 1990

Printed and bound in Great Britain by
HarperCollins Publishers Ltd, Glasgow

Preparing for Pregnancy

Professor Geoffrey Chamberlain is Chairman and Head of the Department of Obstetrics and Gynaecology at St George's Hospital in South London. He has worked in the Royal Navy, the Postgraduate Medical School and King's College Hospital. He was a Consultant Obstetrician at Queen Charlotte's and Chelsea Hospitals for many years and after private practice became a Professor. He teaches medical students, midwives and postgraduate doctors, and has performed research on fetal development and the care of women during pregnancy and labour.

Professor Chamberlain is married to another medical professor and they live in Wimbledon. Their five children are now in the reproductive phase themselves and so far there are six grandchildren.

Contents

Foreword

Professor Geoffrey Chamberlain is well known nationally and internationally as an academic, a practising obstetrician and an author. With these talents and his energies combined it is not surprising that the result is an excellent book which fills a long recognized gap. For a decade or more the profession has declared its interest in prepregnancy counselling yet relatively few centres have been developed to undertake this very important work.

By the time the average mother-to-be sees her medical adviser the initial formative process of the developing embryo has taken place. If ever we are to make any impact on the early development of the embryo and advise about the risks to maternal and fetal health we must encourage parents-to-be to come for advice before pregnancy starts.

This book gives good advice to would-be parents explaining, with Professor Chamberlain's usual clarity, the reasons for seeking advice and the ways in which prepregnancy counselling can be of help. It gives good advice on health education for this very important time in a woman's life, and by its clear explanations sets out to dispel many of the myths and anxieties which concern prospective parents. The text is very explicit and does not shy from discussing the more difficult and tragic complications which cannot be totally avoided. The factual information given is helpful and his innovative offer to answer any questions posed to him on the tearaway slip at the back of the book is, like the author himself, more than generous.

This is a book which would-be parents should read, but also members of the profession who are not involved in

prepregnancy counselling would do well to catch the enthusiasm in Professor Chamberlain's message.

Sir George Pinker, KCVO
Royal College of Obstetricians, London
1990

Preface

This volume is written for those who have doubts. Many wonder about a forthcoming pregnancy; they are concerned about what may happen and sometimes have worries they do not wish to discuss in the open. Others are concerned about specific points before they get pregnant, perhaps the influence that previous illness or lifestyle may have on the unborn child. In addition, a growing number of people wish to prepare for pregnancy; they want to know about certain aspects of living that may be changed before pregnancy starts. Based upon the author's experience of many years in running prepregnancy clinics, this book offers information and advice for all these groups of people.

I am most grateful to two women who wish to remain anonymous who, having been inpatients in St George's Hospital for many weeks, were kind enough to read through the whole typescript, pointing out many areas where they felt changes in the writing would make it clearer. Their comments have made the volume more helpful to the reader and I am grateful to them for the time they gave me. My thanks are also due to Duncan Larkin, the medical artist at St George's Hospital, who drew the black and white illustrations so skilfully, to Anne Fraser who has typed the various drafts with great skill, and to the Fontana editors who have been so helpful at all stages, Alex Howell, Kelly Davis and Juliet Van Oss. I am of course grateful to Culpeper for his forthright writings which provided most appropriate quotations to head every chapter but one. For the exception I have taken the liberty of reading between Culpeper's lines and saying what I think he would have said.

One point of style may require explanation: the masculine pronoun has been used throughout when referring to the unborn child. This is simply for convenience (to avoid the unnaturalness of 'it' and the clumsiness, when used frequently, of 'he or she'). I hope it will cause no offence.

I would be happy to answer any questions about prepregnancy that any reader would care to send me, using the question slip printed at the back of the book. This may be removed without spoiling the sequence of the book and sent to me at St George's Hospital, Cranmer Terrace, London SW17 0RE.

Finally I would like to thank the thousands of couples who have come to me for advice over the years. It is their experience that I have learnt from and that I set down here in order to try to help others in the future.

Geoffrey Chamberlain
St George's Hospital, London

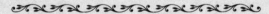

Nicholas Culpeper was a herbalist in the
seventeenth century. He wrote a very popular
*Guide for Women in Their Conception, Bearing
and Suckling of Children* which was first published in 1651 and had seventeen reprints until
1777. This was an important volume for it
covered prepregnancy care as it was known 300
years ago. Quotations have been taken to head
each chapter – the forthright instructions given
are indicative of the age in which Culpeper
lived.

Section I

INTRODUCTION

ONE

Why Take Prepregnancy Advice?

Your child is nourished by your own blood,
your blood is bred by your own diet rectified
or marred by your exercise, idleness, sleep or
watching. Nature sees and knows how you
swerved from what is fitting.

Culpeper

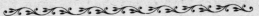

Having a baby is a natural process requiring no thought and little preparation. So run the ideas of those who drift from one event in life to the next, accepting the cards that nature deals and doing nothing to lessen the odds. In the Western world, virtually nobody follows a *laissez-faire* philosophy like this now. Most women will turn for help to midwives and doctors during the birth of the child, the time of maximum need. At this late stage medical help can only provide emergency treatment, salvaging babies from damage during birth. Many women, even the most ardent nihilists, now go further, realizing that preparation for childbirth must take place in the lead-up period; so they present themselves for antenatal care to their doctor or clinic. In the Western world, 98% of women now go to antenatal clinics, where treatment is aimed at preventing problems in the mother or her unborn fetus.

However, a growing number of couples wish to prepare for childbirth before this stage. If antenatal care can help the growing of the unborn child, would it not be sensible to prepare for pregnancy by ensuring that the parents are in the best state of health before conception? This is the essence of prepregnancy care, a concept which has been in the background for many years and about which ideas have been crystallizing in the last decade.

In 1920, Janet Lanecoop Plaipol wrote in *The Child Welfare Movement*:

> The teaching of all the experiences in child welfare work was to throw back further the need for care from

the period after birth to the period before birth and then, yet further, to help the woman before marriage.

Antenatal care started at the beginning of this century in Edinburgh and developed slowly until the 1920s. One of the tenets of good antenatal care is early attendance. Pregnant women are urged to see their family doctor as soon as they think they are pregnant and ideally, he refers them to the antenatal clinic so that their booking visit takes place in the first few weeks of pregnancy. However, this does not actually happen very often. Most women in the United Kingdom book for antenatal care at eleven to thirteen weeks of pregnancy.

In a recent survey at a big London hospital, it was found that women having their first baby had realized they were pregnant on average five and a half weeks after their last menstrual period or ten days after their missed period; among those who had had a child before, this recognition time was reduced to four and a half weeks or a couple of days after the missed period; there was obviously a range in the numbers of women occurring on either side of these averages. These figures indicate that women know they are pregnant – and could act on this knowledge – long before the conventional times when they go for medical care.

The improvement in and wider use of pregnancy tests in the last decade has allowed such early suspicions to be confirmed. Few women, however, excepting those who have had a problem in the past, attend an antenatal clinic earlier than eight to ten weeks after the first day of the last normal menstrual period.

One of the major avowed purposes of early antenatal care is to help women avoid influences that might cause malformations in their child. (This is dealt with in more detail in Chapters 2 and 3.) Most fetal abnormalities occur in the first ten weeks of pregnancy; after this, the fetus continues to grow but the organs have already been formed. Therefore, in these first important weeks, it is wise for a woman to avoid the obvious hazards which might cause an abnormality in the embryo.

Known examples are X-rays, the taking of certain drugs, and infection by some viruses such as German measles. Yet, since most women start antenatal care after these first ten weeks, they often arrive too late to influence malformations. A little time spent at a clinic before pregnancy could inform a woman of these very important aspects of early pregnancy and advise her how to avoid certain dangerous situations.

The advantage of prepregnancy consultation is that it allows a wider range of options. If it is left until pregnancy has started and problems are then detected there is only one choice open to a couple – either the pregnancy continues regardless or a doctor may be able to offer a termination. If the pregnancy continues, then the couple must accept the consequences of any problem in the growing embryo. If they decide not to continue with the pregnancy, and there are reasonable grounds of higher risk, an abortion can be performed but this is a traumatic choice even for those who agree with abortion in theory; when it comes to having an abortion oneself, thoughts sometimes change. Further, there are many people to whom abortion is anathema; they may live in countries where it is not even an option. In the light of such difficulties, it is better to discuss such problems before pregnancy starts when there is no pressure and time allows for a wider series of options to be considered.

If a woman comes for prepregnancy advice, she may be offered many alternatives; for example, if she has a long-standing disease which might affect the growing embryo, she can be counselled about the course of that disease, its natural progression or the way it may be improved by treatment. This might allow gaps to be identified in phases of the disease when the couple could think of starting a pregnancy. Such a series of remissions is found frequently in certain conditions such as ulcerative colitis*. Again, a disease process might require the woman to take drugs continuously; these themselves may be dangerous to the fetus. By discussion with her and the physi-

*Words marked thus are referred to in the Glossary.

Case Study

Mr and Mrs A W did not meet until he was fifty-two and she forty-three. Working together, they fell in love and decided to marry. When Mrs A W was forty-four they thought they would like a baby and while she was vaguely aware that older women had a more difficult time, her mother had told her this was a question of her frame of mind only.

She wondered whether to seek medical advice before getting pregnant but a holiday in Morocco intervened and so the first time she consulted a doctor she was twelve weeks into her pregnancy. He advised her about the various problems of pregnancy in her age group, including a consideration of the risks of Down's Syndrome or mongolism. Mrs A W was horrified; she had not appreciated this was an age-related condition and so requested an amniocentesis*. This could not be done until sixteen weeks had elapsed and the result came back at nineteen weeks of pregnancy. Unfortunately, it showed that the baby she was carrying had Down's Syndrome. After much anguish Mr and Mrs A W requested termination of pregnancy which was performed at twenty weeks.

When they were told that the risk of a Down's Syndrome baby in her age group was 1 in 40, both Mr and Mrs A W were adamant they would never have started a pregnancy with odds like that. They wished they had gone for prepregnancy advice, for it would have saved them many weeks of anguish.

cians looking after her, it is often possible to reduce or change these medicines for a few months to allow a pregnancy to start and establish itself at a time when the mother is taking no drugs.

A woman's condition may be so severe that the chances of producing a live baby are remote. Adoption might be one solution for this couple. In the United Kingdom at the moment, adoption is very difficult, for there are few babies available. There are still some, however, who can be adopted under certain circumstances. If the couple belong to the Catholic church, for instance, there may be a number of babies available, as the Abortion Act of 1967 has made little difference to the beliefs of mothers following certain religions and abortion is still unusual. Many blame the generally low numbers of adoptable babies on the 1967 Abortion Act for in the last twenty years the number of pregnancies terminated in the early weeks of gestation has increased from a few thousand a year to over 170,000. Whilst some of these babies would have been kept by their mothers it is probable that many would have become available for adoption had the option of abortion not been made so easy in England, Wales and Scotland. In 1967, the year that the Abortion Bill was debated in Parliament, about 23,000 babies were put up for adoption in this country. Twenty years later in 1986, the number was only 472 under six months, while another 7,400 older children who had been fostered first were also available. This is an enormous reduction in the numbers of babies available for adoption in this country.

Consequently, potential parents are looking to adopt children from other parts of the world. In the 1970s they went to the Far East but now many countries such as Thailand have altered their laws about the adoption of their nationals by foreigners to make it more difficult for Europeans to adopt children. At the moment many adopted children come from South America; the precise number is unknown, but one agency in Peru reported that it negotiated and made the arrangements for the adoption of 300 children into the United Kingdom in 1989 while the smaller country, Israel, adopted at least 2,000 Brazilian babies. Finding children overseas, however, is a difficult and tortuous business, costing a great deal of money and involving complex medical and legal consultations. For many couples it is not the alternative to having a pregnancy themselves.

If there were to be a hereditary problem on the male side, some couples could turn to artificial insemination. For example, if the husband of a Rhesus negative woman was himself

Rhesus positive, in certain circumstances all the sperm he made would carry Rhesus positive chromosomes. Since this is a dominant gene, each baby he fathered would be Rhesus positive. With each child the degree of severe Rhesus* effect would be increased so that the babies would eventually not survive pregnancy and be stillborn.

Until recent advances in Rhesus treatment made it possible to deliver such children alive, the only hope for such a couple was to conceive and produce a Rhesus negative baby. This is not possible with the husband but could be done by artificial insemination with sperm from a Rhesus negative donor. The egg (the oocyte) would come from the woman and she would carry and give birth to the child so many couples would feel that the child was truly their own.

An extension of artificial insemination – egg donation – is undoubtedly going to come to the Western world in the next decade. Already many cases of this have been performed, for, while it is frowned upon by many societies, it is not yet illegal in most countries. Opposition is not logical, for if one accepts artificial insemination by donor sperm, philosophically one should support artificial impregnation of a donor egg.

In such a circumstance, the husband's sperm fertilizes an egg from another woman *in vitro*. The resulting child would be genetically half his, half the donor's. The fertilized egg would be inserted into the uterus of the man's wife thirty-six hours later. Pregnancy would result and in time the wife would give birth, making the baby very much a part of the family.

Not all problems can be circumvented at a prepregnancy clinic. Often the couple have a potentially uncorrectable problem and they wish to know the odds of hazards in pregnancy or the degree of effect on the unborn child even though nothing in medicine can be done to change these chances. These risks can usually be worked out based on what has happened to other couples who have suffered the same combination of circumstances previously. This is not a perfect matching process, for no couple is exactly like another, but it gives an indication of the zone of risks so that the odds can be considered. This book contains many incidences of such risk figures and when they apply, the couple should discuss them individually. Some may then feel that the risks are too high and so they may decide to remain childless; they would settle down to use contraception or even seek the permanency of sterilization of the husband or wife. This is a voluntary decision made with deeper knowledge given at the prepregnancy clinic.

Case Study

In the days before we could test for cystic fibrosis* in the amniotic fluid, Mrs W F came to see us in the prepregnancy clinic. She already had one child aged two and a half who was moderately affected by the condition and wanted to know about the chances of its recurring in another pregnancy. With the help of a geneticist, we worked out a fairly specific risk which we told her and her husband. She thought about this and then went into the next pregnancy accepting these odds. She felt much happier in the pregnancy, knowing that the risks were slight.

The end result was a happy one for she gave birth to a child who was not affected by cystic fibrosis. Mrs W F felt much happier in pregnancy knowing what the chances were rather than going through with a vague, nagging doubt throughout the whole of her pregnancy.

However, a note of caution should be sounded. With the recent advances in genetics (see Chapter 4), it is possible that in the next few years many conditions now thought to be incurable and untreatable will be corrected by genetic manipulation using recombinant DNA therapy. Hence, it would be wise in some instances for couples not to consider sterilization unless the advice of a consultant geneticist has been obtained. He or she may know that just over the horizon there is some research which could bear on this couple's problem and that it is likely to come to fruition within the next few years. Permanent sterilization should be postponed in these circumstances.

These are some of the reasons for seeking prepregnancy advice in relation to specific diseases or family histories. Total prepregnancy care, however, should obviously form a part of the way we live; looking after oneself in the time before an embryo is implanted in the uterus and during early development gives a special incentive to learning more about a balanced lifestyle. Ideally, we should always eat a proper diet, refrain from excesses of tobacco and alcohol, take exercise, and use only prescribed medicines in minimum quantities. This is all commonsense, but it stands out in sharper profile at a time when a new baby is being formed and starting life inside the uterus. So much of prepregnancy care is an extension of the general tenets of living healthily. Unfortunately, in the urban Westernized society in which many of us spend our lives, we have forgotten these tenets and they need reiterating. The prepregnancy period is a particularly good time for this.

Prepregnancy care can be seen in three tiers, like the wedding cake that symbolizes the start of many marriages. The bottom layer is the general advice which should be available to everybody at all times of life. It should be given in schools and youth clubs and is probably best absorbed as part of the general biology of living, a subject rarely taught in the secondary schools in the United Kingdom but widely lectured on in other countries, such as Japan. The media are now becoming increasingly interested in health matters and articles and programmes help to spread knowledge.

Supported on the first tier, the next layer of prepregnancy care would be for couples who wish to take advice on specific subjects. For example, the woman may be a school teacher wondering about the hazards of German measles to which she is exposed each year from her pupils. Such a specific problem can be best dealt with by a variety of medical helpers, but the advice is individual to that couple. It may be that the family doctor can give the best advice for he or she knows their background and often has a knowledge of the woman which no clinic doctor can achieve. Further, the family doctor often has a less formal relationship with the couple and they may be happier to see him or her rather than go to a hospital clinic. Family doctors can also check the woman's blood pressure and if they think it relevant, do other blood tests such as that for the haemoglobin* level to check for anaemia*. They may reinforce the advice about general problems such as smoking and alcohol, and thus perform a useful part of the prepregnancy service.

As well as the family doctor, family planning clinic doctors may be familiar to the couple or they may prefer to consult a health visitor they know. In some parts of urban Britain, relationships have been struck up very strongly between the population and the hospital direct. This is so in South London and at St George's we offer an open access prepregnancy clinic in the evenings, run by one of our sister midwives who is knowledgeable in these matters and talks informally with couples.

The top tier of advice, supported by the other two, is the specialist prepregnancy clinic; to this come couples with specific medical problems. These may relate to diseases already present, potential genetic problems because of family history, or problems relating to previous pregnancies. Such cases require obstetricians who, as well as their knowledge of pregnancy and childbirth, specialize in maternal medical diseases in obstetrics. These include the effects of disease and its treatment on the unborn child. They must have close links with colleagues in genetic counselling and the capacity to find out information rapidly when they do not know the answer. This is one of the hardest things for doctors to admit; some never do, for they feel they should always present a front of omnipotence to those who consult them. People attending the prepregnancy clinic, however, are not patients but couples who want information; rather than give vague or misleading answers, the doctor should admit he or she does not know of certain unusual combinations of factors and then go and find out. Nobody minds this attitude; it is one that the author has used for thirty years without any apparent harm or loss of confidence.

Special prepregnancy advice clinics are now available in many parts of the Western world. They have usually been set up by those who have an enthusiasm for the subject, and the family doctor will know the nearest one. He or she is therefore the best person to consult when one wants advice for a specific medical problem. In the United Kingdom, prepregnancy clinics have been set up for special conditions such as Rhesus* disease or diabetes.

The first general obstetrical prepregnancy clinic in the UK started at Queen Charlotte's Hospital for Women in January 1978. It was an informal consultation clinic to which most couples came by referral from their General Practitioner although self-referral was not refused. At the clinic, the obstetrician would allow about half an hour for each couple's appointment, for this is an area that cannot be hurried. It is important that both partners attend since each often has different aspects of problems to discuss. Further, they can later reinforce to each other what was said.

It is often found at the prepregnancy clinic that the problem outlined in the General Practitioner's referring letter is only the beginning of a series of problems which are discussed. The obstetrician at the clinic must be able to tease out these problems and discuss each one of them separately with the couple. If the answers are not immediately available, then the couple is offered a second visit in a few weeks' time so that reports of past medical events can be obtained from other hospitals or more precise information about the conditions can be discussed. In some clinics, an examination of the woman is offered; at others, it is performed only occasionally depending upon the nature of the problem. Some simple blood tests may be done, again depending upon the problem, but it should be emphasized that these clinics are orientated towards specific problems which the couple brings to the prepregnancy clinic. They are not general health clinics; for these, the couple should consult their family doctor.

Conclusions

Prepregnancy care is not a new idea. The concept is based upon general health education concentrating on this one special time in life. However, this time zone is particularly important to couples and it is right that a small number of doctors concentrate their attention on it. Most of the advice given for general health applies at the period prior to pregnancy, but there are other special aspects worrying couples for which there should be expert advice available. Not everybody is close to a specialist prepregnancy clinic, nor does everybody want one, but for those who need it, a short journey may bring them into contact with experts who can advise them on those aspects of a forthcoming pregnancy that might worry them. Many obstetricians working in district general hospitals perform the same function without formally setting up a clinic. If a couple want specific advice, a General Practitioner can usually obtain an appointment with an interested obstetrician locally who would be prepared to offer a consultation and go into the details of the problem. He or she would give answers that have the strength of being relevant to the local facilities available. Thus the couple would have the benefit of relevant prepregnancy care even without a formal clinic in their locality.

Armed with such advice and having discussed previous worries, the couple can either be shown how to overcome their problems and make a plan for the future or they can face these problems squarely and make rational decisions about whether or not to proceed with a pregnancy.

Section II

THE GROWING EMBRYO

TWO

What Happens Normally in Early Pregnancy

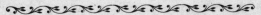

In the act of copulation, the woman spends her seed as well as the man, and both are united to make the conception.

The seeds of both sexes being united, the womb instantly shuts up, partly to hinder the extramission or passing out of the seed, partly to cherish the seed by its inbred heat, the better to provoke it to action . . . then instantly nature goes to work.

Culpeper

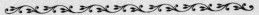

The embryo starts to lay down the structural foundations of the child's future body in the first days of pregnancy; it is therefore important to consider this time before going onto the complexities of growth and organ formation. We all started as a single cell, a result of the fusion of a sperm and an egg. From that, we multiplied within a few weeks to make a fetus composed of six billion cells, a rate of growth and cell division faster than at any other time in life.

Fertilization

The Egg
The eggs (or oocytes) are made in the ovaries, a pair of walnut-sized, solid organs on either side of the woman's pelvis. All the eggs for future fertility are stored here. The ovaries also produce large amounts of the female hormones, oestrogen and progesterone, which act in the body in a cyclical way to give the woman her female characteristics.

The eggs come from several million individual cells laid down in the ovary before the woman was born. Unlike a man, a woman has a finite number of cells that can turn into eggs, while a man can go on making new sperm throughout his life. The woman produces eggs from the age of fifteen to forty-five approximately, whereas the man can produce sperm from puberty to over seventy years of age. The woman's fertile time is limited to about thirty years, whereas the man's is more elastic, for some sperm can be made even in old age.

The two million or so primitive eggs with which the woman is born reduce rapidly in number during infant life; by the time she reaches puberty there are probably only half a million left. These mature at each menstrual cycle so that each twenty-eight days a potential egg is prepared for possible fertilization. If day one is the first day of menstrual bleeding, by the sixth day of the cycle, most women with regular periods will have produced a series of minute fluid-filled cysts which start to swell in the ovary; each cyst contains a primitive egg. Probably several hundred start the process but very few grow past 2 mm (⅛ in) in diameter; the others stop developing and are absorbed back into the body. Those left swell so that by the tenth day, there are only four or five at the 5 mm (¼ in) stage, and by the twelfth day, one or two have reached 10 to 12 mm (about ½ in) in diameter. On day fourteen, when one of the follicles*

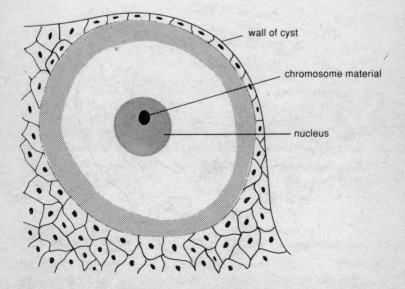

wall of cyst

chromosome material

nucleus

Figure 1 The ripe egg which is shed from the ovary on day fourteen of the cycle. The nucleus contains a half complement of chromosomes and genes for passing on to the future child after fertilization.

has usually reached about 20 mm (¾ in) in diameter, the wall of the cyst on the outer side of the ovary gives way and a blob of jelly containing the primitive egg is squeezed out (see Figure 1). This microscopic egg contains the nucleus with the mother's half of the chromosomes for the potential child. All the other eggs which started in the same cycle and did not reach the final stage of development have been absorbed; they play no part in reproduction.

The process of egg shedding continues every month throughout most women's reproductive life so that by about forty-five years, there are no more eggs left in the ovary and a woman can no longer have babies. The hormone cycles will continue for a few years more with the pituitary gland releasing hormones which attempt to stimulate the ovary more and more forcibly in an effort to release eggs. Eventually it is obvious from the hormone feedback from the ovary that there are no more eggs

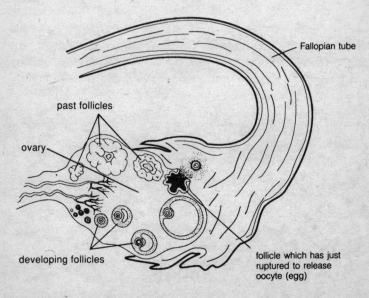

Figure 2 The open end of the Fallopian tube embraces the ovary to collect the egg as it oozes out.

to be produced and the hormone stimulation by the pituitary gland reduces; with that menstruation stops, leading to the menopause.

The egg produced in each fertile cycle appears on the surface of the ovary on about the fourteenth day of a twenty-eight-day menstrual cycle. The outer end of the Fallopian tube usually surrounds the ovary so that a veil of finger-like protrusions embraces the blob of mucus on the ovary, and the egg travels straight into the Fallopian tube (see Figure 2). When it arrives there, it rests in the wider, outer end of the tube. If fertilization is going to take place, the sperm will travel up to meet the egg here.

The effective life of an egg is about thirty-six hours and that of the sperm a little less. Fertilization is possible therefore for only a day or so in the middle of the menstrual cycle. On all the other days of the month, there is no egg available and so intercourse will not result in fertilization. The 'safe period' is based on this principle, used by those preferring the natural family planning methods of contraception. Conversely, this knowledge of timing is also used by those attending fertility clinics and who wish to have a baby. You can time this method more precisely by the techniques outlined in the Box below.

Checking the Time of Ovulation

Most women have a menstrual cycle of twenty-eight days. Usually one egg is produced in each menstrual cycle; if it is not fertilized it is absorbed and the uterine lining is shed so that menstruation follows fourteen days later. Hence, a woman with a regular twenty-eight-day cycle ovulates fourteen days before menstruating. Since the cycle is twenty-eight days long, ovulation must be fourteen days after the first day of menstruation, i.e. mid-cycle. However, if a woman has a thirty-five-day cycle the fourteen days from egg production to menstruation is still constant. Ovulation will therefore occur twenty-one days from the beginning of the previous menstruation.

The time of ovulation is reasonably precise in women who have a twenty-eight to thirty-day cycle, give or take a day. If the cycle is irregular other methods must be used. These are:

Basal Temperature Charts
In the second half of the cycle, after the egg has been produced, the hormone progesterone causes the body to work slightly harder so that the total basal temperature is slightly raised. By taking the temperature every morning before getting out of bed and plotting it on a chart for two cycles, the slight temperature rise can be detected.

Blood Tests
A blood test done in the latter half of the cycle can show a raised progesterone level. This confirms that an egg has been made but will not pinpoint the time of ovulation.

Checking the Cervical Mucus
During most of the menstrual cycle cervical mucus is thick and tacky, like Gloy glue. However, for one or two days around the time of ovulation it becomes very thin and streamy. A sensitive woman can detect this by gentle examination of her own vagina.

Lower Abdominal Pain
A very small number of women get a lower abdominal pain lasting four to six hours at the precise time of ovulation. This may be more to one side than the other and is felt sharply for an hour or so, gradually fading away. It is caused by a little fluid surrounding the egg spilling into the peritoneal cavity. If a woman notices this pain then she knows very precisely when ovulation has occurred, but not all women get it.

The Sperm

The sperm start their life in the testicle of the father where they are mass produced in enormous numbers all the time, not just during sexual arousal. After travelling in tubes from the testis to a storage sac at the back of the prostate gland, the sperm rest for some weeks while their nuclei are maturing.

At the time of ejaculation, a jet of fluid passes from the prostate gland into the male urethra; as this column of fluid is travelling rapidly down the urethra, a bolus of sperm is injected into it from the storage sac. The sperm-rich semen then rush on through the penis and are ejaculated into the upper vagina at the climax of intercourse.

On average a man produces well over a hundred million sperm at each intercourse. These are highly active, single-cell organisms, each with a head containing the nucleus with half the chromosome material for any future baby (see Figure 3).

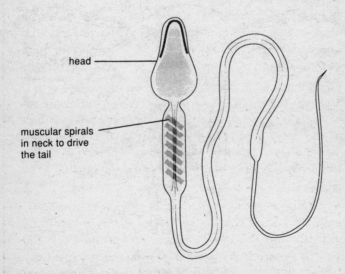

head

muscular spirals in neck to drive the tail

Figure 3 A sperm, the head of which contains half the complement of chromosomes for the future child. Behind the head, the neck is joined to the long, whipping, active tail.

The head is capped by a slightly pointed area, the acrosome, containing enzymes which can help tissue penetration. Behind the head is a muscular tail containing a series of nine spindles running its full length; by contraction of these in a programmed fashion, the tail propels the sperm in a corkscrew way, passing through fluid at immense speeds.

Only a little of the semen ejaculated into the upper vagina around the cervix ends up at the entrance to the uterus near the opening of the cervix in the vagina – the external os (see Figure 4). The sperm in that area progress up through the cervical canal towards the uterus. At the time of ovulation, their passage is helped by a change in the complexity of the cervical mucus, a plug of which usually guards the canal. The mucus is composed of a tangled skein of molecules, rather like coils of barbed wire in an army encampment. This prevents bacteria and other micro-organisms rising from

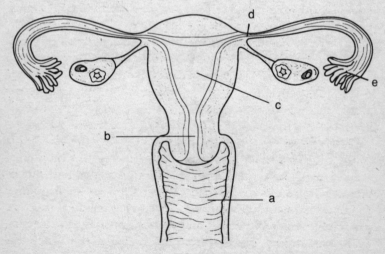

Figure 4 The journey of the sperm from upper vagina to the outer end of the Fallopian tube takes thirty to forty minutes. Deposited in the upper vagina (a), those sperm which may perform fertilization travel up through the cervical canal (b) into the uterine cavity (c). A few reach the inner end of the Fallopian tube (d) and swim out at the far end (e) where an egg may await them once a month.

the vagina to the uterine cavity and so keeps the latter sterile. For a day or two around ovulation, however, the barbed wire strands straighten out, making lanes like a swimming pool in the Olympics. Thus, the passage of sperm is facilitated at the time of ovulation, whilst the cervical mucus acts as a relative barrier for the rest of the menstrual cycle.

The remaining sperm – some 99% of those ejaculated – stay in the vagina and travel in random directions, hitting the side walls of the vagina or the recesses around the cervix. Some semen trickles down the vagina when intercourse is over and the penis is removed. This is perfectly normal and the loss of semen from the entrance to the vagina occurs in most women. This is not related to any reduction in fertility, for the semen escaping contains those sperm that would never have been strong enough to enter the uterus anyway. Those sperm which are going to be effective for fertilization have already travelled into the cervical canal and passed through it almost before intercourse is concluded.

The sperm pass between the organized molecules of cervical mucus into the cavity of the uterus where they travel in all directions on the surface of the endometrium* which lines the uterus. Only a few thousand arrive at the top of the uterus where the Fallopian tubes leave. The Fallopian tubes are each 10 cm (4 in) conduits, joining the cavity of the uterus to the sides of the pelvis where the ovaries lie. Normally, the lining of the tube is thrown into many folds covered like the pile of a carpet with hair-like filaments (cilia) beating on the surface and causing a current of fluid to pass from the outer part of the tube towards the inner end. This helps any fertilized egg progress towards the uterus and in addition acts as protection against ascending infection from the vagina to the abdominal cavity. Another mechanism which helps the egg on its way is the Fallopian tube peristalsis, a wave of muscle contraction passing down the tube from the outer end to the tube's opening into the uterine cavity. This action milks down anything floating in the fluid, reinforcing the action of the cilia. Conversely, at the time of ovulation, there is a reduction or even reversal of action of these two current-making facilities. The cilial action is suppressed while the peristalsis is stopped or even reversed, so helping the passage of sperm from the uterus to the outer end of the Fallopian tube.

The sperm enter the Fallopian tube, travelling mostly in the valleys between the folds, for there are fewer cilia here to oppose their action and the currents are even more sluggish. With their rapidly lashing tails propelling them along, and the lack of peristalsis against them, the sperm soon reach the outer end of the Fallopian tube, the first getting there within thirty minutes of intercourse. Although the distance may seem small – about 15 cm (6 in) – body size to body size it is equivalent to a 180 cm (6 ft) man running from London to Brighton in half an hour. That is an impossible athletic feat, yet it is performed every time sperm travel through the woman's genital tract. During the course of this journey, the numbers of sperm are greatly reduced; of the hundred million that started in the upper vagina, a few hundred only will arrive around the egg.

Fertilization
The egg and the sperm thus arrive at the same point in the body. The egg gently floats in body fluids rotating in an anti-clockwise direction; those sperm that have completed the long journey, swim round it. One of them penetrates the outer coat of the egg and within minutes, a biochemical reaction produces an ionic barrier in the outer cell membranes which means that no other sperm can penetrate. The sperm which does penetrate is nipped off behind its nucleus, its tail left wriggling outside the egg. The nucleus of the sperm, containing the father's half of the chromosomes of the future baby, migrates towards the nucleus of the egg containing the mother's half of the chromosome complement. Nuclei fuse and the chromosomes pair off together, thus for the first time making the new individual with a unique set of forty-six chromosomes, ranged in twenty-two pairs plus a pair of sex chromosomes. If there are two X chromosomes, a girl will result. If there is an X and a Y chromosome in the pair, then a boy will be born. The time

of sexual determination is at the moment of conception and nothing after that can change it.

Each sperm bears the potential for making a boy or a girl. Most men produce roughly equal numbers of male-making and female-making (androgenic and gynogenic) sperm, although a few may produce a slight preponderance of one over the other. The various manoeuvres that people try to ensure they have a child of the sex they desire are outlined in the Box below. None of them are very effective and despite claims made, few stand up to any scientific proof that they predetermine the sex of the forthcoming child significantly. However, if people wish to try to change their luck after a series of two or three babies of one sex, they may attempt some of the non-harmful methods indicated.

Having a Boy or a Girl

Producing a child of the desired sex is a very basic human wish and goes back several centuries; many of the current myths date back to the ancient Greeks.

In folk lore the right side of the woman's body is considered to reflect masculinity and the left side femininity. Aristotle believed that the right ovary produced males, whilst Hippocrates advised the husband to bind up the right testicle before coitus if he wanted to produce a son. From these ideas come a series of tales of the woman's position during or just after intercourse helping to produce a child of the desired sex.

The sex of the child is determined by the husband's sperm; those which carry male-making chromosomes are sometimes more active and move faster than those bearing female-making chromosomes. In consequence, in artificial insemination in other species it has been possible to separate these two sorts of sperm outside the body by physical means. That part of the sample containing

---

(Having a Boy or a Girl cont.)

the higher concentration of those sperm producing the desired sex has then been used in artificial insemination. This has been tried in humans without any great success.

Some people try to alter the acidity in the vagina, for this may affect the activity of the sperm. Male-making sperm favour a slightly more acid environment. Hence, gels with a slightly more acid background are introduced into the vagina; in theory more male-making sperms will get through and so progress up to the cervix. This method does not give very precise results because those sperm which are going up as far as the egg stay in the vagina for a very brief time after ejaculation.

Dietary measures have also been recommended to produce male children. It is alleged that if a man stays on a certain seafood diet for eight weeks, at the same time abstaining from intercourse with his wife, he will be more likely to produce a male child. There is no scientific evidence that this works.

Passage through the Tube

The fertilized egg starts its journey down the Fallopian tube, propelled by a gentle current. The single cell (see Figure 5a) starts to divide after twenty hours into two cells; the new nucleus elongates and forms a dumb-bell, nipping off the middle, making two nuclei, each containing a full complement of forty-six chromosomes. This is followed soon by a new cell membrane growing across the middle, so two new cells are produced (see Figure 5b). After a few more hours, these two cells divide to make four and then eight cells (see Figure 5c); after ninety-six hours, this has grown into a multicell clump (see Figure 5d). Meanwhile the egg, a structure with no means of propulsion, is wafted down towards the uterus in a current of fluid, whipped up by the cilia, on the tips of the ridges of the tubal lining and by gentle peristalsis of the muscle of the Fallopian tube.

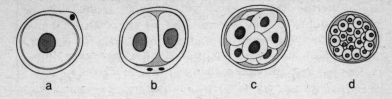

Figure 5 Cell division of the egg from one to two cells to many cells. A *morula* (mulberry) of cells is formed by about the time the egg reaches the uterus. This soon forms a hollow sphere with the embryonic disc at one pole.

The clump of cells now resembles a miniature mulberry (see Figure 6a). Some of the cells inside the berry are not in contact with the fluid which bathes the fertilized egg in the Fallopian tube. This fluid provides all the oxygen and nutrients for the rapidly growing cell bunch and takes away the waste products that the cells produce, an effective transport and exchange mechanism for the cells on the outside of the clump, but not very helpful to those inside. They have to pass their oxygen and nutrients one way and the waste products the other through the outer cells. A cleft appears in the middle of the *morula* (Latin for mulberry) of cells, so that most cells are near the surface where nutrient exchange occurs (see Figure 6b). The cleft fills with fluid (see Figure 6c) so that by the time the fertilized egg arrives in the uterus, some seven days after fertilization, it has become a hollow sphere (see Figure 6d).

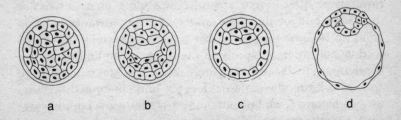

Figure 6 Development of the solid ball of cells into a hollow sphere to ensure that all cells have contact with the surrounding fluid.

The uterine lining is soft and ready to receive the egg. The hormones of the second half of the menstrual cycle have prepared the lining and much nutrient material is already stored. The hollow *morula* settles on the surface of the uterus (see Figure 7a) and hormones from the surface cells help it to burrow down into the uterine lining. The egg settles down within a couple of days so that it is almost completely hidden from the cavity of the uterus on the tenth day after fertilization (see Figure 7b). Limb-like projections of cells branch out from the surface of the egg in order to anchor the clump of cells; they also provide a bigger surface area, for all nutrition is now received from the mother's blood which surrounds the egg, but does not enter it. Rapid development occurs in the next few weeks so that most of the organs have been made by the end of ten weeks and the embryo is anchored in a sac of fluid by the umbilical cord whilst exchange with the mother's blood supply is occurring through the placenta.

The Development of the Organs

The Brain and Spinal Cord

About sixteen days after fertilization, a ridge of cells running down the length of the primitive embryo thickens and grows rapidly. This then sinks below the surface of the disc and becomes a trough. The edges of the trough join and seal off the cavity so making a tube, with the overlying skin closed over it (see Figures 8a/b). The sealing process starts at the lower end of the body and moves up towards what is going to become the head. This tube is to become the spinal cord and it expands rapidly in the head; being limited by the overlying skin, growth can only occur by kinking the tube and convoluting the surface. Thus the brain is formed, with its unique pattern. Two buds of the neural tube grow rapidly sideways to make the specialized human upper brain containing its many cells and interconnected pathways. In the next twenty weeks, very rapid growth will occur in this organ so that most

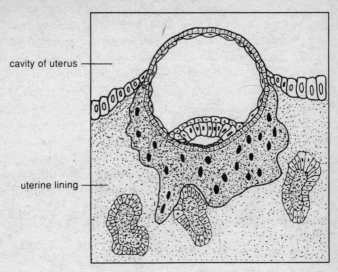

Figure 7a Implantation of the fertilized egg into the uterine lining.

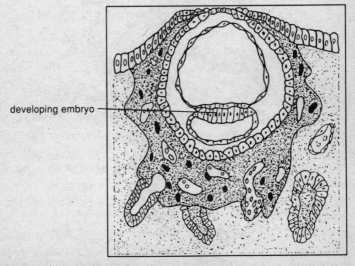

Figure 7b As the embryonic body cavities develop, the whole structure sinks into the maternal tissues and draws nourishment from the surrounding blood.

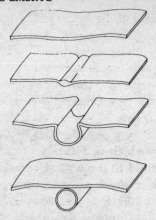

Figure 8a The brain and spinal cord develop from the valley of skin that sinks into the tissues to form a tube.

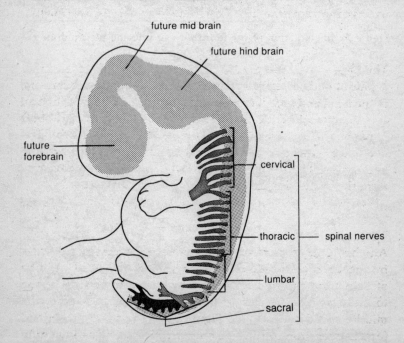

Figure 8b The brain end enlarges rapidly and folds over. The nerve protrusions grow out from the developing tubular nervous system.

of the cells of the brain of the future individual are already laid down halfway through pregnancy. After that, growth occurs in the intercellular substances and the insulating material that covers all the pathways inside the brain.

The rest of the neural tube passes down the back to become the spinal cord from which nerve protrusions are sent out. These are long channels of tissue, each connected to a cell in the spinal cord; they group together in clumps to form the nerves of the body which in future will carry the sensations from the outside world to the central nervous system and the motor responses from the brain or spinal cord, travelling in reverse direction, to the muscles. As the limbs and organs grow, they carry these nerves with them to regulate coordination in the various parts of the body.

The spinal cord and brain are well formed by about eight weeks of intrauterine life. Further development is by growth.

The Eyes

A pair of buds of nervous tissue from the brain passes forward in the head end on either side of the future nose (see Figure 9a). As it approaches the overlying skin, the end of each bud is pushed in to form a cup of two layers (see Figure 9b). The overlying skin sinks onto this cup and forms the lens and the eyelids (see Figure 9c). The two layers of the cup themselves form the retina and the supporting coats of the eye.

The Ears

Another pair of nervous-tissue projections passes sideways from the brain substance to each side of the head. A tube of skin from the future throat grows upwards on each side to meet a pocket of skin at the side of the head to form the middle and outer ears (see Figure 10a). The tissues meet and form the ear drum, whilst the outgrowth of nervous tissue from the brain produces the inner ear, with its hearing and balance sensations (see Figure 10b). The outermost part of the organ, which most of us recognize as the external ear, is formed by a series of skin projections around the pocket which sink in to form the ear drum. Later in embryonic life, cartilage forms in these skin folds to stiffen the external ear.

The Limbs

At first the embryo is a simple cylinder but by twenty-eight days the head has grown rapidly because of brain growth and eyes are beginning to appear. Just before the fifth week of intrauterine life, the limb buds appear, the arms just behind the head, and the legs halfway up the body (see Figure 11). These are tubes of skin filled with poorly differentiated tissues; as the skin buds grow the tissues follow, differentiating into bone and muscle.

When the limbs have reached a certain length, joints appear in the future wrists, elbow and shoulder of the arm, and knee, ankle and hip of the leg. Around these joints ligaments condense to strengthen them so that they do not dislocate. At this early stage, the joints are only gaps between the bone and the limbs in which bending can occur, but soon a more sophisticated arrangement develops. The two bone surfaces which engage upon each other have complementary shapes and on this surface a smooth layer of cartilage is laid down. Thus the shoulder joint becomes a ball and socket while the knee becomes a hinge joint. Cartilage is a self-lubricating, smooth tissue which, as it wears away, produces more cells. The smoothness of all the joints of the body depends on this self-reproductive principle.

The ends of the limb buds flatten into discs in which the small bones of the hands or feet differentiate like the ribs of a fan. At first, the fingers and toes are joined together; they separate later, leaving a small web of skin between each. On the back surface of the tips of the fingers and toes, cells thicken and sink deeper making a horny layer which grows forward as a nail.

Along the limbs grow the nerves which come from the

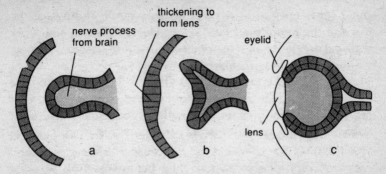

Figure 9 The developing eye: Nerve protrusions grow forwards from the brain towards the skin (a). They become eggcup-shaped while the skin in front of them thickens (b). The skin sinks in to form the lens and eyelids, while the nerve protrusions make the inner light-receptive surface and the outer layers (c).

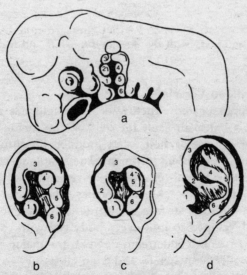

Figure 10 The external ear develops from the primitive gill folds: in (a) they are arranged circumferentially around the ear orifice. In (b) and (c) the pattern becomes more convoluted, and (d) shows the position of these gill remnants on the new-born baby's ear.

spinal cord. They link with the sensory nerve endings of the skin and the motor plates in the muscles. The hand, being our principal organ of fine sensory discrimination, has an extremely rich nerve supply to its skin.

Limb movements start from eight to nine weeks of embryonic life and can be seen readily on ultrasound scanning just after this time. The mother, however, does not usually feel such movement until sixteen to twenty weeks of gestation.

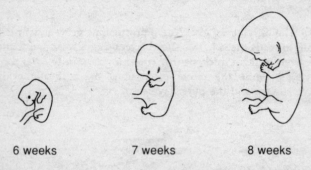

6 weeks   7 weeks   8 weeks

Figure 11 Limb buds with the developing hands and feet.

Blood and Blood Vessels

Once the sophisticated structure of many cells has developed as the embryo it is difficult for cells on the inside to obtain nutrients or dispose of their waste products by diffusion with the surrounding fluid environment. The simple mechanism of making a hollow ball of cells, as the more primitive *morula* did, is not efficient any more. Most of the tissue layers can no longer be in touch with the surface so an internal circulation of fluid has to be developed to link every body cell with oxygen and food supplies. The bloodstream flows in the major blood vessels and smaller branches to and from all tissues in the body so that every cell at the periphery of the body communicates with the great blood vessels in the central trunk. To circulate this volume of blood requires an efficient pump which will drive blood to the organs and limbs, allowing it to flow back to the centre for reoxygenation and another supply of nutrients before being pumped out again. The simple circulatory system of heart – placenta – heart in the fetus, changes at the moment of birth into heart – lungs – heart – body – heart in the adult.

In the blood are numerous red cells which carry oxygen to the tissues; these float in the fluid plasma containing many proteins and other food substances going to the cells. Four weeks after conception islands of blood-forming cells are found in various parts of the body. Groups of cells lining these areas branch off to form blood vessels. The cells in the centre of the islands make red blood cells. Those float away in the fluid which becomes the plasma.

All the arteries and veins grow rapidly with the developing tissues, passing down the limbs and to the organs as the tissues are being laid down. Running the full length of the embryo are a pair of big arteries with one-way valves. The muscular walls of these thicken sharply in the chest region (see Figure 12) and start a regular pumping action from about twenty-three days after conception. This propels the blood in one direction and so starts the circulation. The tubes grow rapidly and, since they are held permanently at each end, they bend and kink into compartments. The lining develops with folds at the angles of the kinks between the compartments of the heart. Soon the four-chamber heart of the adult has been formed with bypass mechanisms to allow for the non-functioning lungs in the fetus.

When the fetus is *in utero*, oxygen and blood come from the placenta so the flow patterns of the bloodstream are modified. After birth, blood on the right side of the heart is pumped to the lungs where it is oxygenated and returned to the left side of the heart. From there it is dispersed to all the tissues of the body. In the unborn child, the lungs are superfluous organs which are bypassed by blood flowing through an incomplete partition between the two sides of the heart. At birth this hole usually closes when lung circulation is established but occasionally it stays open and the child remains with a hole in the heart. This leads to an inefficient circulation of oxygen, so the blood is less pink and the child is slightly blue (cyanosed). Previously, such babies did not live long but now cardiac surgery can easily close such holes and the baby can lead a normal life.

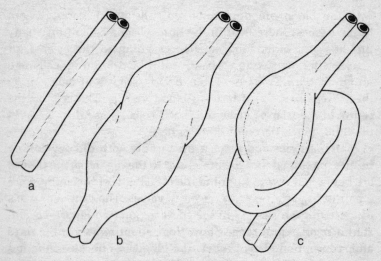

Figure 12 The development of the heart: (a) A pair of simple tubes conducting blood. (b) In places the wall thickens to provide a muscular pump which creates a fluid current. (c) Growth is rapid; the tube, fixed at each end, becomes convoluted to produce the heart as we recognize it.

Digestive Tract

Once the embryonic organs are organized, nutrients are no longer diffused through the surface cells. Distribution now takes place through the bloodstream which picks up nutrients and oxygen from the placental exchange system and passes them to the fetus cells. Meanwhile, the digestive tract has to develop so that immediately after delivery, when the placenta is separated, a baby can switch to oral feeding and absorption of all nutrients needed from the intestine.

In the embryo, the intestine comes from an elongated tube

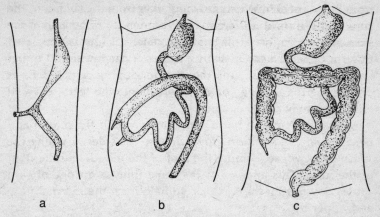

a   b   c

Figure 13 Development of the stomach and intestines. The relatively simple tube (a) grows rapidly and, being fixed at each end, convolutes. It also dilates in places to become the stomach and large intestine (b and c).

running the length of the baby; this communicates at the head and tail end with pits of skin that sink in from the face and anus respectively. The gut tube grows more quickly than the body around it and can only find space by twisting (see Figure 13). The tube is suspended from the back of the embryo's body; as it twists loops occur. Some parts enlarge in diameter as well as in length, forming the stomach or the large intestine. The muscle rings in the wall of the tube thicken in a few places to make sphincters, such as the pylorus at the exit from the stomach. The stomach itself enlarges greatly and this allows us to feed at intervals, taking in more than we immediately require but then allowing us freedom from eating for several hours while the food is kept, partly digested in the stomach, being released in small amounts to the digestive tract. From the walls of the gut tube, buds of tissue grow out to form the eventual liver and pancreas.

At the head end, the gut tube comes into contact with a piece of skin that sinks in from the face. The pit of the tube joins the mouth cavity with the gut (see Figure 14). The lips develop from bulges of skin which grow together from the sides and the jaws come from undifferentiated, hardened tissue under the skin in the form of cartilage at first; later calcium is deposited to form bone. On the matching ridges of the lower and upper jaw, small pits of skin sink into the developing cartilage. Later on, these produce pegs of very hard bone, the teeth, covered with extremely dense enamel.

At first the embryo has a common space for the mouth and nose but soon a platform grows in from the sides, dividing the space into two, so forming the roof of the mouth and the floor of the nose. This appears at the same time as a ridge of skin comes down from the forehead to help form the external nose and upper lip.

At the other end of the body, the gut tube joins another pit from the tail skin which forms the anus. This zone is surrounded by muscle rings that form the protecting sphincter to control the passage of faeces.

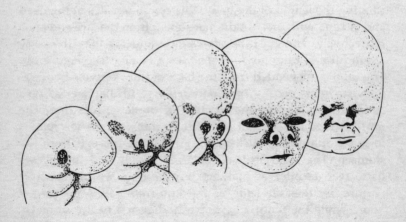

Figure 14 Development of the face. Over three weeks the face is formed from a series of folds which grow in from the sides and fuse. These are shown in the first four diagrams. By fourteen weeks, the face looks human, although the proportions are different from those of an adult.

The Genital Organs

The genital organs consist of the gonads that make the sperm or eggs and the passages that conduct these germ cells or gametes to the outside world. In the woman these are the Fallopian tubes, the uterus, cervix and vagina, whilst in the man the passages are the vasa deferens, running from the testis to the seminal vesicles, and the urethra which leads from the back of the prostate gland through the penis. All these systems develop in close association with the urinary tract.

The gonads arise from a pair of ridges on the back of the abdominal cavity whilst the tubal systems are left over from remnants of the urinary tract evolution. The gonadal tissue starts swelling at about five weeks in the region of the kidneys and is drawn down towards the pelvis. During this time, male or female gonads develop.

If there is a Y chromosome present, testicular differentiation takes place, stimulated by a series of sex-developing enzymes. If there is no Y chromosome, then the embryo develops as a female. Being male involves having testes following the presence of a Y chromosome. Being female involves not having testes, whether the ovaries are present or not. Testicular function is determined by the presence of androgens (hormones like testosterone) and inhibitors of the development of ovaries. (The ovaries are present in the early life of every embryo and would develop unless testosterone stopped them.)

Without the presence of a Y chromosome, testosterone levels are low and so gonads develop into ovaries. These adhere to the back of the membranes surrounding the future uterus and there develop the primitive eggs discussed earlier. If testosterone stimulation has caused the gonad to develop into a testis, it is drawn into the inguinal canal* and then passes down in the following weeks to reach the scrotum. Occasionally, its advance is slow and many boy children are born with the testis in the canal or at its entrance, not having fully entered the scrotum.

The testis can be distinguished by about seven weeks when

a large number of sex cords develop which will produce the sperm. The ovary cannot be identified positively until some time later. The primitive germ cells (those that are capable of becoming eggs) form under the surface and by twenty weeks, they have reached several million in number.

The vagina develops from a common bud of tissue below the bladder and in front of the rectum. This is a solid rod of tissue in the female, and by sixteen to eighteen weeks of embryonic development, the central core breaks down to form the lumen of the vagina. It joins onto the remnants of the primitive renal drainage system which has formed the uterus and Fallopian tubes.

In the male, the lowest part of the lower abdominal wall grows out to form the primitive penis. The bladder drains into the tip of this protuberance of tissue while erectile tissues grow into it from the pelvis.

Growth

Most of the changes in the developing organs and limbs take place by ten weeks of pregnancy. Hence, most congenital abnormalities have occurred by this time; thereafter development is by growth, so that few defects can start after these weeks. This is important because many women are uncertain whether or not they are pregnant in the first weeks of gestation, and by the time pregnancy is confirmed it is often too late to take precautions, for fetal abnormalities may already have occurred.

The embryo grows very rapidly during pregnancy, particularly in the middle months. No limb or organ will ever grow as rapidly as this again, for if the speed of growing were to continue at that rate until later life, after twenty-one years the child would be as tall as Nelson's Column and weigh as much as a heavy army tank. Growth rates slow up considerably after birth (see Figure 15).

Different parts of the body grow at different rates. The blood which is richest in oxygen is conducted to the embryo's head so that the brain and head grow quickly. The embryo looks big-headed and indeed at birth a normal child's head is much larger in proportion to its body than people are used to seeing in older children. This, and their slight baldness, makes babies appear rather like Winston Churchill.

The limbs of the embryo have little use inside the uterus so they have a relatively poor blood supply. They are small and look puny at birth. Even in the first few months after birth, human babies do not use their limbs for weight-bearing so growth is still slow. Once an infant starts to crawl, however, the legs become stronger and grow longer in proportion to the body.

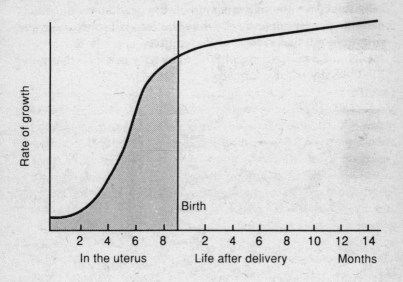

Figure 15 Growth of the fetus is most rapid in the middle three months of pregnancy and then tails off to a rate which will be maintained in infant life after birth.

Conclusions

Nature produces many more eggs and sperm than are needed for the natural process of replacing the species. There are enormous odds against any given sperm meeting any egg; on such chance couplings are based our genetic futures. The egg after joining with the sperm travels to the uterus along the Fallopian tube; many fertilized eggs do not complete that journey but are absorbed. Once safely implanted, the egg elaborates the organs of the body rapidly from about sixteen days after fertilization to about fifty-five days. The brain forms and grows from a simple tube to become a convoluted computer of intercommunicating cells served by the nervous system, the heart starts to beat as early as twenty-three days, while the face is formed from the primitive gill-like system of the embryo. The rate of development is most rapid in this phase and by ten weeks of intrauterine life the baby is fully formed.

THREE

What Might Go Wrong with the Embryo?

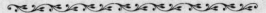

The imagination of the mother operates most forcibly in the conception of the child. How much better then were it for women to lead contented lives, that so their imaginations may be pure and clear, that so that their conception may be well formed.

Culpeper

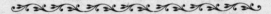

Congenital abnormalities are structural deficiencies of organs and limbs produced in the fetus during his life in the uterus. Some congenital defects are obvious immediately after birth; others are not diagnosed for weeks or even years after delivery. The more serious abnormalities are usually discovered very soon after birth, for they affect the life and wellbeing of the child.

In Britain, of every thousand born, between ten and twenty-five babies have an abnormality. Some are serious such as heart disease; others are less so like skin tags in front of the ear which do not present a life-threatening problem. Higher rates of abnormalities are found amongst babies who do not survive the full length of pregnancy. Many embryos miscarry in early pregnancy and modern research indicates that two-thirds of embryos expelled before the twelfth week of gestation have either a chromosomal or structural abnormality. These embryos cannot cope even with intrauterine existence and certainly would not have survived outside the uterus. This is nature's way of preventing too many abnormal children being born.

Abnormalities

The Causes of Abnormality

Abnormalities may have one of two causes. Either there is a genetic problem with an inherited alteration in the chromosomes, or else some environmental cause has acted directly on the early embryo. The former problem includes both the familial inherited abnormalities, such as cleft palate and hare lip, and mutations which occur in the chromosomes from either egg or sperm, for example Down's Syndrome occurring in the older mother. At present it is impossible to take any action against these types of abnormality. Prepregnancy counsellors can discuss the odds of their happening but cannot prevent them. However, with advances in DNA technology, gene manipulation is rapidly becoming possible. This has already been carried out in some animal species so that in the future it may be possible to remove the gene sequence causing the problem, replacing it with a normal group of genes which will allow the future child to lead a normal life.

If identifiable, environmental influences might be avoided. They include: infections (such as German measles); drugs (such as thalidomide); physical injuries (such as X-rays); oxygen deficiency (such as indifferently given anaesthetics); and nutritional deficiency (such as absence of vitamins). All these are possible to identify and then avoid.

Many of the environmental causes act at a specific time when organs or limbs are at their phase of maximum differentiation or growth. The hazard does not have the same effect before or after that time and the specific time zones are fairly narrow in fetal life. For example, the spine may be affected between five and six weeks of development but is unlikely to be affected at other times. Similarly, problems may come in the upper limb from five to six weeks while those in the lower limb come from six to seven weeks. The heart is most likely to be affected from five to seven weeks of development and the alimentary tract varies from the upper end (five to six weeks) to the lower end (six to seven weeks). Most organs are formed by ten weeks and few congenital abnormalities can therefore start after that.

Prepregnancy counselling is useful in this area to help sort out a couple's reactions to congenital abnormalities. If there has been a family history of an abnormality, prepregnancy advice may help determine whether this is environmental or genetic. If the couple had a previous baby with an abnormality, again the cause can be sought and sometimes found. Unfortunately, however, most abnormalities seem to arise out of the blue with no obvious cause. Learning from those who attended prepregnancy clinics, we might be able to identify more reasons for some abnormalities and thus avoid them in the future.

Common Abnormalities Around the Time of Birth

This next section is not meant to worry potential parents but to explain what the abnormalities are, how they are caused and what can be done about them.

THE NERVOUS SYSTEM

Anencephaly
Incidence: 1 in 400
Occasionally a baby is born with no development of the brain. Anencephaly is incompatible with life and most affected babies are born dead. The cause is not known but some believe it may be associated with a lack of vitamins at the time of conception combined with a genetic tendency towards this condition.

Spina Bifida
Incidence: 1 in 600
A spina bifida is a defect in the skin or muscle of the back over the lower spinal cord. In Chapter 2, details were given of the trough of skin which sank in from the back and the fusing of the skin over it. A baby with a spina bifida has suffered from a deficiency in the skin and muscle fusion. In consequence, varying amounts of the spinal cord are exposed to the outside. In some, the skin may have fused but the underlying tissues have not, and so a thin sac is spread over the spinal cord tissues.

Spina bifida may be detected antenatally by ultrasound at sixteen to eighteen weeks or a suspicion of an open spina bifida (one with no skin cover) may be confirmed by a raised level of alpha fetoprotein in the mother's blood tested in the antenatal clinic at sixteen weeks. The presence of spina bifida rarely interferes with delivery; it is wise that the baby is seen by paediatric surgeons and neurologists very early. Sometimes spina bifida defects can be closed early and treatment can lead to a happy conclusion. Much depends on how far the nerve supply to bladder, anal sphincter and lower limbs is permanently damaged. Unfortunately, neither the alpha fetoprotein levels nor the extent of the defect seen on ultrasound can predict the degree of damage. Many parents therefore wish the pregnancy to be terminated in view of the lack of precision in the prognosis.

THE BONY SYSTEM

Talipes
Incidence: about 1 in 700
The baby has one or both feet turned inwards. This position might be related to tight intrauterine pressure on the feet; it cannot usually be diagnosed before delivery.

Usually the deformity is not serious and corrects itself. If not, early physiotherapy and strapping gives a good result. In extreme cases, surgery may be required later in infancy to correct the angle of the foot to the shin. This is unusual.

Dislocation of the Hip
Incidence: 1 in 600 amongst girls
          1 in 2,500 amongst boys
Dislocation of the hip is usually an isolated malformation although it may be associated with spina bifida. It is more common in breech presentations. All babies have their hips examined immediately after birth to check there is no dislocation. If this condition is diagnosed, the infant should be seen early by an orthopaedic surgeon.

Commonly, a simple splint will keep the head of the femur in the socket of the pelvic bones and, with the rapid growth of early life, the child's hip position is rectified. Problems occur if congenital dislocation of the hip is not diagnosed before the child starts to bear weight when he crawls and later starts walking. Then the dislocation becomes a chronic condition and, once it has become established, treatment is very difficult. If diagnosed early, treatment of hip dislocation is straightforward.

Phocomelia and Amelia
Incidence: 1 in 30,000
Amelia is a complete absence of the limbs, while phocomelia is a shortening of the arms or legs. This rare abnormality was brought to prominence by the thalidomide outbreak in the 1960s; if that drug was taken at a precise time of limb development, arm or leg shortening could occur. There are usually no other abnormalities of the rest of the body and no deficiency of mental development. Such abnormalities are very rare now that thalidomide has been withdrawn from use among women in the reproductive age.

Extra Digits
Incidence: Very common
Extra digits may be found on the hands or the feet. This is commonly a familial trait and may involve a complete extra finger or a small skin tag containing a little cartilage on the border of the hand or foot. Occasionally this is associated with fusion of other fingers so that the web between the fingers is higher up the finger or toe gap than usual.

If there is just a skin tag on the edge of the hand or foot, it can be tied off with a nylon thread in the neonatal period. If cartilage is present in this extra digit, more formal surgery is required and is usually postponed until later in the infant's life.

URINARY SYSTEM

Absence of Kidney
Incidence: 1 in 500

This is usually not diagnosed in early life, for the child appears perfectly normal. When later in life, examinations are performed for other reasons, the absence is noted.

There is no treatment for this and many people with a single kidney lead perfectly normal lives, never knowing about the absence of the second organ.

Valves in the Urethra
Incidence: 1 in 5,000–8,000

These are folds of tissue in the tube passing urine from the bladder to the outside. They can cause obstruction so that the bladder becomes enlarged and then back pressure may damage the kidneys. Usually they are diagnosed in the neonatal period; with ultrasound they can be suspected while the baby is still in the uterus. Treatment is by surgical removal of the folds; this should be prompt in order to avoid long-term back pressure on the kidneys causing damage.

Hypospadias
Incidence: 1 in 200

The orifice of the penis may not be quite at the tip of the glans but a little behind it. This leads to difficulties in the direction of the urine in later life. It is important that such a child be seen by a paediatric surgeon reasonably soon. Under no circumstances should a circumcision be performed; if surgical correction is required in the first or second year of life, all the skin available may be required for that.

Undescended Testicle
Incidence: 1 in 100 boys

Often the testicle is no lower than the exit of the inguinal canal or is in the canal itself. In these cases, it can usually be brought down into the scrotum by the doctor's fingers. If not, the child should be checked again at a few months to see if the testicle has descended. If still required, a small operation is usually performed at age two or three.

ALIMENTARY SYSTEM

Hare Lip
Incidence: 1 in 400
This condition is very distressing to parents, for the face is the most visible part of the body and is the focus of much emotion. The hare or cleft lip has a familial tendency. The cleft may be one-sided, coming in line from the nostril, or two-sided, coming down from both nostrils. There can be feeding problems and often the hare lip is associated with a cleft palate.

The condition can be surgically corrected, usually within a few weeks, often in the early neonatal period, and excellent results come from this in the hands of good plastic surgeons.

Cleft Palate
Incidence: 1 in 400
The palate extends from the back of the upper ridge of teeth to the throat. A cleft palate may be a small nick in the back of this platform or it can extend to become a complete gap to the front, even including the dental arch. Feeding problems develop and special teats or spoons are required.

Surgery produces good results; this is usually postponed for six to twelve months until the child has grown.

Tracheo-oesophageal Fistula
Incidence: 1 in 3,000
The fistula is an open communication between the windpipe and the gullet. It is usually diagnosed within the first hours of birth, and surgical treatment is urgently required. Babies usually do well after this.

Pyloric Stenosis
Incidence:1 in 400 boys
            1 in 800 girls
There is an increase in the bulk and strength of the muscle at the pylorus, the exit from the stomach. In consequence, milk is retained and the child vomits in a projectile fashion, hurling the milk as much as 0.6 m (2 ft) away. It is commonly diagnosed between one and four weeks of life because of persistent projectile vomiting and failure to thrive. A small operation can divide the enlarged muscle and the child becomes perfectly normal after this.

Upper Intestinal Tract Obstruction
Incidence: 1 in 2,000
The various parts of the intestine may be blocked by lack of proper canalization during development.

The duodenum is a more common site and in a third of cases it is connected with Down's Syndrome. The baby will vomit all food from the beginning. An X-ray usually helps make the diagnosis and early surgery produces good results.

Blockage may occur further down the intestine following damage to the blood supply. In this case a longer time is required to make the diagnosis, for the gut can hold a certain amount of fluid before it is vomited back. These are usually isolated problems and can be successfully treated with surgery.

Lower Intestinal Tract Obstruction
Incidence: 1 in 10,000
This is usually diagnosed soon after birth because no meconium (fetal faecal material) is passed. This is confirmed when the midwife tries to check the baby's first temperature with a thermometer in the bottom and she cannot insert the instrument.

X-rays are needed for full diagnosis; surgical treatment usually produces good results for this problem. In about half the children, the condition can be immediately treated by a simple operation with excellent results. In the remainder a temporary colostomy is necessary until definitive operation at six to nine months.

Another major obstruction in the lower large intestine arises from a deficiency in the nerves which are normally present in the bowel wall (Hirschprung's disease). A temporary colostomy relieves the problem and allows the child to thrive until an operation performed at the age of nine months. The results of treatment are excellent.

Imperforate Anus
Incidence: 1 in 5,000
The absence of an anus should be obvious on first examination of the child. Surgical treatment is needed urgently in this situation; either a colostomy to relieve pressure and allow the stools to pass out, or an operation to make a permanent opening, with muscles, in the region of the anus.

Exomphalos
Incidence: 1 in 4,000
A congenital herniation of the contents of the stomach may occur through the stomach wall if the muscles are missing. The hernia is just covered by a sac and skin and the baby needs urgent treatment in a paediatric unit.

Surgery can correct the immediate deficit but the treatment is over a long term. If a sac is present, the outlook is not as hopeful.

THE CARDIOVASCULAR SYSTEM

Incidence: 1 in 200
Many congenital heart problems are minor; they are now diagnosed more often because of better examination of the newborn in the days after delivery. Treatment is not always required, for, as the child grows, some of the lesser problems correct themselves. Poor oxygenation follows with cyanosis (a blue baby) and a raised pulse or respiration rate. Many heart

problems have no apparent symptoms but a murmur is discovered by the doctor at examination. Sometimes this cannot be heard immediately after birth, for the heart rate is too fast then, but within a few days these murmurs are detected.

Urgent paediatric cardiological opinion is required and special investigations will reveal the degree of the heart lesion. Many of the problems diagnosed can be left under observation and will correct themselves; of the rest, most can be treated simply although a few do require surgical correction.

CHROMOSOME ABNORMALITIES

These malformations are laid down from the time when the chromosomes fuse at fertilization.

Down's Syndrome
Incidence: overall 1 in 800
The incidence is strongly associated with maternal age (see Table overleaf). The rate is very low below the age of thirty, being less than 1 in 1,000; by thirty-five it rises to 3 in 1,000 but by forty it is 10 in 1,000 and increases even more after that. Risk becomes greater with age but the condition can still occur in babies born to younger mothers. The father's age appears to have less effect on this condition than the mother's. It is thought that most cases are due to an extra chromosome in the mother's egg nucleus which joins with the sperm at fertilization. Hence, there will be three chromosomes in position 21; the condition is known as Trisomy 21* (see also page 68).

Down's Syndrome is usually diagnosed at birth, for the child looks slightly mongoloid. He will have upward-slanting eyes, which are rather small. The folds on the inside of the eye are pronounced whilst the head is generally flattened with diminished front-to-back diameter. The ears are low-set and the nose is small with a flat nasal bridge. The mouth is also often small and the tongue protrudes from it, while the neck is short and broad.

The Risks of Down's Syndrome by Age

Maternal Age (years)	Risks of Down's Syndrome
30	1/880
31	1/820
32	1/720
33	1/600
34	1/460
35	1/360
36	1/280
37	1/220
38	1/180
39	1/140
40	1/100
41	1/85
42	1/70
43	1/50
44	1/40
45	1/30
46	1/25
47	1/20
48	1/15
49	1/12

The hands have stumpy fingers and only have one crease on the palm instead of the usual two. The skin is dry and the baby often seems limp. Such babies have a higher than usual incidence of associated abnormalities of the heart and obstructions of the bowel. These, however, can usually be treated with surgery.

The main problem with Down's Syndrome is mental retardation later in life. This does not show in the newborn period but, as the child grows, the mind lags behind the body. This is a very variable feature and not one upon which any prognosis can be given at birth. Some children achieve a mental age of four or five by the time they are physically in their teens; others may not do quite as well as this.

Down's Syndrome and other chromosomal abnormalities

can be diagnosed in the antenatal period. Either a chorionic villus biopsy may be made at ten to eleven weeks of gestation when a small fragment of the edge of the placenta is removed for microscopic examination, or cells shed from the fetus are recovered at sixteen weeks from an amniocentesis when fluid is withdrawn from the uterus. One of these tissues can be cultured and the chromosomes examined to detect Trisomy 21 or other faults. A new series of biochemical tests is being developed for Down's Syndrome: a series of hormone and protein markers in the blood of mothers of all ages can be assessed at sixteen weeks to give a suspicion of Down's Syndrome and so indicate the need for an amniocentesis. This is available only at a few hospitals at present.

Edward's Syndrome
Incidence: 1 in 2,000
This condition is also associated with an extra third chromosome on the position of chromosome 18 (Trisomy 18*). The baby is born with a small head, the back of which is prominent and beaked; there are also often malformed ears, a cleft palate and talipes of the feet. Heart and intestinal defects are common and often there are deficient kidneys. Survival is not long with Edward's Syndrome.

Turner's Syndrome
Incidence: 1 in 2,500 girls
This is not usually detected in childhood, although occasionally the fact that the baby has a short neck and low hairline leads paediatricians to make a diagnosis. There is an absence of a second sex chromosome, so the chromosomes are designated XO. In later life, these girls have short stature and problems with ovulation.

These are the major chromosomal problems seen at birth. There are many other, more severe conditions, but these are so disruptive to life that the embryo does not survive and a miscarriage occurs in the early months of pregnancy.

It should be recalled that all the abnormalities in the United Kingdom only make up 1 to 2% of births and therefore most women have a 98% chance of giving birth to a baby without an abnormality. The risks of each is listed below.

Incidence of Abnormalities

Anencephaly	1 in 400
Spina bifida	1 in 600
Talipes	1 in 700
Dislocation of the hip	1 in 600 girls
	1 in 2,500 boys
Phocomelia and amelia	1 in 30,000
Extra digits	very common
Absence of kidney	1 in 500
Valves in the urethra	1 in 5,000-8,000
Hypospadias	1 in 200
Undescended testicle	1 in 100 boys
Hare lip	1 in 400
Cleft palate	1 in 400
Tracheo-oesophageal fistula	1 in 3,000
Pyloric stenosis	1 in 400 boys
	1 in 800 girls
Upper intestinal tract obstruction	1 in 2,000
Lower intestinal tract obstruction	1 in 10,000
Imperforate anus	1 in 5,000
Exomphalos	1 in 4,000
Cardiovascular system	1 in 200
Down's Syndrome	overall 1 in 800 (*see table on p.56*)
Edward's Syndrome	1 in 2,000
Turner's Syndrome	1 in 2,500 girls

Conclusions

Up to twenty-five out of every 1,000 babies born in the United Kingdom have some abnormality. Many of these are small and have no effect on future life; others are larger, requiring diagnosis before delivery so that appropriate care can be given immediately after birth. With such a problem, women are best delivered in large hospitals where all the facilities for caring for the child can be met immediately.

Abnormalities might be due to problems in the formation of the chromosomes. Most genetic programmes are laid down at the time of fertilization, but a few may be altered in the young child. Other abnormalities may be caused by environmental influences acting on the embryo at the time when the early tissues are dividing. These include physical and chemical damage as well as infections, and can be identified and so avoided.

Section III

THE COUPLE'S BACKGROUND

FOUR

Genetic and Chromosomal Influences

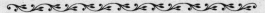

Men and women beget men and women, then
if their hearts be not united in love, how should
their seed unite to cause conception?

Culpeper

Much of what we are is inherited from our parents. Millions of genetic messages have been transmitted from the nucleus of our parents' egg and sperm to the next generation in the chromosomes which have been inherited from our father and mother. These develop as the embryonic body grows inside the mother's uterus; the chromosomes are strands of protein molecules arranged in special sequences to send genetic messages from one set of cells to the next, controlling structure and function. At reproduction, one set of messages comes from the father and another from the mother. They merge mostly but some are occasionally dominant over others.

In all cells, there is a nucleus filled with dark material; this is mostly made up of coiled strands of chromosomes. When uncoiled, they are shown to be forty-six pairs of strands specific to our species. Other species have different numbers of chromosomes; some fern plants have as many as 1,000 pairs of chromosomes. The chains are intermingled so that on microscopic examination they appear as a dense, dark mass, but if the human cell nucleus is broken open and analysed when cell division is occurring, the strands may be teased out into the twenty-three pairs of autosomal or ordinary chromosomes of different lengths.

In addition, are the sex (X or Y) chromosomes. As explained on page 27, these determine the sex of the baby.

At specific places along the length of the chromosome, the inheritable signals are sited. The genetic information is stored on nucleic acids which make up two chains of molecules of phosphates and sugars joined together by specific combina-

GENETIC AND CHROMOSOMAL INFLUENCES · 65

tions of the chemicals purines and pyrimidines. When the sugar
is deoxyribose, the nucleic acid is known as deoxyribonucleic
acid or DNA. Other nucleic acids involve the sugar ribose and
so are called ribonucleic acids or RNA.

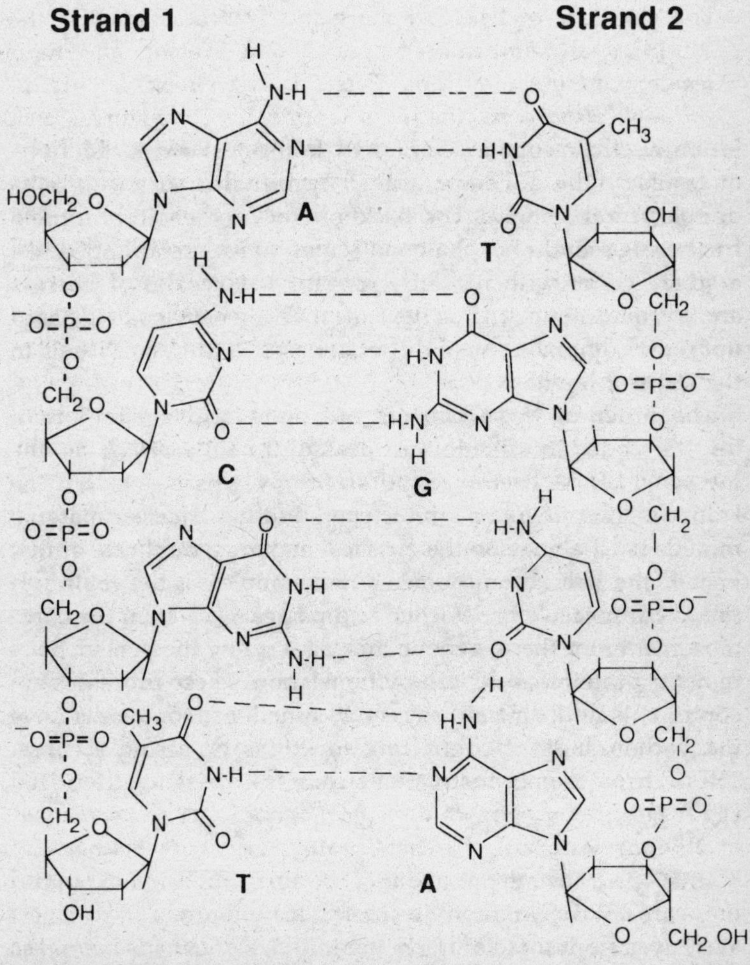

Figure 16 Chromosomes are made of long strands of DNA molecules
linked by bands. When chromosomes divide, the bands (shown by
dotted lines) separate, making two strands.

This differentiation is of more than chemical interest. DNA is found in the chromosomes and makes up the basic storehouse of inherited characteristics. RNA is the message molecule which carries the signals from the DNA out to the rest of the cell nucleus for implementation by cellular activity.

The structure of DNA in the genes was calculated in the early 1950s at Cambridge by Crick and Watson and their research won them a Nobel Prize. It is well written up in *The Double Helix*, a fascinating scientific detective story which is eminently readable. Crick and Watson showed the DNA molecule to be a compound of two chains arranged in a double spiral or helix. The backbone of each chain is formed by the sugar and phosphate molecules which are arranged like a spiral ladder with regularly repeating molecules of purines and pyrimidines acting as the rungs. The genetic code is based upon the combinations of different bases* at different levels in the steps of the helix.

The order of these clusters of amino acids is important for the code. Information is passed from the DNA to the messenger RNA by transcription. Briefly, this means that the ladder is undone like a zip fastener, and new nuclear material moulds itself alongside the zip face, making a duplicate of that part of the half chromosome. When completed, the replica of the DNA molecule is detached and passes away from the chromosome. From there, genetic messages go by messenger RNA to other proteins in the cell by translation. These processes are continuous and control basic body functions; some cells have many thousands of controlling functions occurring at once. These chromosomal instructions come to the newly fertilized egg.

Obvious instances of genetic traits passed from father and mother to a baby are the colour of the eyes, the hair and height; these are not the product of a single gene but probably of several. They are but three of the many millions of genetic messages that pass from the parents at the fusion of the two gametes when fertilization occurs. The genetic programme is thereby laid down for ever in that new individual. The expression of genetic messages may be modified by environmental factors later and these twin influences control the future development of the baby. Whether the environment can influence genetic transmission over the next generations is debatable. It is partly implied in Darwin's *Origin of Species* but the process might just be one of more efficient reproduction among those better fitted for a new environment rather than one of changes being built into the genetic code.

Genetic Disorders

The consideration of inherited problems forms an important part of prepregnancy care. Genetically caused changes occur in all families; most are normal, but a few cause major structural or functional congenital abnormalities such as a cleft palate. As more environmental hazards are being understood and limited, genetically determined abnormalities are becoming relatively more important. About 1.5% of liveborn infants have a genetic congenital abnormality. Although some of these conditions are lethal at birth, this group makes up one-third of the admissions to the paediatric wards. In addition, many of the common diseases of adult life have a partial genetic component, such as coronary heart disease, cancer or diabetes. As will be seen later in this chapter, 50 of every 1,000 live births have a detectable genetic problem which can affect the quality of life.

Geneticists divide genetic disorders into four groups: chromosomal abnormalities; single gene disorders; multifactorial disorders; and disorders with a partial genetic component. Perhaps someone in the family has had a congenital disease or, just as worrying, someone says there is some vague history of a relative who had a problem. If this worries you, read on.

Chromosomal Abnormalities

These are gross abnormalities in the number or the structure of chromosomes; they can be seen using the light microscope when the chromosomes in a nucleus are analysed. The seriousness of chromosomal abnormalities may be judged by a gradient of effect on the growing embryo; 1 in 200 newborn babies have a chromosomal disorder but 1 in 20 stillborn babies and 1 in 2 embryos who are miscarried early in pregnancy show chromosomal abnormalities. Thus these abnormalities are responsible for serious malformations which do not even allow the baby to survive inside the uterus. They are best divided into abnormalities of the ordinary (or autosomal) chromosomes and those of the sex chromosomes.

AUTOSOMAL ABNORMALITIES

The major abnormalities in this group are due to having either too many or too few whole chromosomes. The most common one is caused when the pair of chromosomes that normally occupies the twenty-first position gains an extra chromosome so that there are three instead of two – a Trisomy 21*. Two chromosomes, instead of one, come from a parent and are joined by a third chromosome from the other parent at fertilization. Trisomy 21 is better known as Down's Syndrome*, which used to be called mongolism.

The extra chromosome material of Down's Syndrome is usually, but not always, from the mother. In a small number of cases, it comes from the father, but this does not bear any relation to the father's age. In the mother, Trisomy 21 is age-related. The risk of Down's Syndrome increases sharply after the age of thirty-five so that by the age of forty, 1% of mothers may produce babies with this condition.

Down's Syndrome is associated with mental deficiency in the offspring. While this may not show at first, as the children grow they fall behind the normal behaviour patterns of development so that after two years it becomes obvious that they are retarded. They can eventually develop a mental age of about six, but there are great variations in individuals and parental care can modify many of the afflictions. Children with Down's Syndrome are very affectionate and families live happily together, caring for the weaker child. There is a higher incidence of heart defects and intestinal obstructions in babies with Trisomy 21. Both are

---

Case Study

Mrs J M had been married four years and had already had two children, aged three and one. She was now thirty-seven years old and busy building up her business as a screen printer, wanting to get on with her life and postpone having a further family. She reckoned it would take five years to reach a position where she would be able to leave her business for long enough to have a baby.

She came to the prepregnancy clinic and we discussed these ideas with her. We gave her the odds of Down's Syndrome occurring in the next few years. These are:

Age	Odds
37	1:220
38	1:180
39	1:140
40	1:100
41	1:85
42	1:70
43	1:50
44	1:40
45	1:30

Mrs J M thought about these and decided it was not in her family's interest to postpone having a baby. She put her business interests to one side and became pregnant; she had an amniocentesis with a normal result and produced a normal third child. Having three healthy children, she and her husband elected to go for sterilization by vasectomy. Last year she started back at work on her screen printing and is already achieving a modest national reputation.

capable of surgical repair and give good results but there is at present no effective curative treatment for the mental defect.

Very few women with Down's Syndrome who grow to adulthood actually have children themselves. If they did, theoretically 1 in 2 of these babies would be affected, for half of the eggs would still have two chromosomes on position twenty-one after division. In fact, most such embryos are miscarried and so far fewer babies affected with Trisomy 21 are actually born.

The converse loss of a whole autosome seems to be lethal in early embryonic life, so that the birth of a baby is very rare. There may, however, be some structural alterations to the autosomes where exchange of a part of one chromosome takes place; when a fragment of one chromosome sticks to another strand this is known as translocation. In others, a segment has been lost and not replaced as happens to chromosome 5 in *Cri du Chat* Syndrome, when the baby's cry sounds like the mewing of a young cat. Many varieties of these abnormalities occur and they can involve any chromosome. An increasing number of rare structural deficiencies is being related to translocations.

The mother and father can be checked, but chromosomal problems occur only in the eggs or sperm; hence there is usually no evidence of such problems in the mother's or father's blood tests although there may be chromosomal abnormalities in their gametes' chromosomes at the time of division. At a prepregnancy clinic, the precise chromosomal translocation cannot be determined from the parents if the previous chromosomal change arose in a single egg or sperm; only karyometric examinations* performed on tissue from a previous baby or miscarriage can show this. Many translocations can be carried in a balanced form in families; here accurate analysis and prediction is possible. Even in the absence of this, parents can obtain useful information about the likelihood of recurrence. The testing of the next fetus in early pregnancy is considered later in this chapter.

SEX CHROMOSOME ABNORMALITIES

As well as in the autosomal chromosomes, abnormalities of the sex chromosomes can occur. These are when extra X or Y chromosomes are associated with the normal sex chromosome. Several varieties of abnormality have been found, such as the Klinefelter Syndrome where there are forty-seven ordinary chromosomes and then an XXY. This usually causes the man to be sterile. In other cases three or four X chromosomes have been found (XXXY). Children are sometimes mentally retarded but occasionally chromosomes are fused so that the excessive number is not apparent. Amongst men, XYY chromosome combinations are rare (1 in 1,000). Such men are often considered to be mentally abnormal and to have criminal tendencies but frequently they are merely impulsive.

Among women, the absence of a sex chromosome (XO) causes Turner's Syndrome in 1 in 2,000–4,000 cases; there are abnormalities of the neck and maybe of the major blood vessels of the body. The woman is usually sterile, for she does not ovulate naturally and so does not menstruate; she is short and has increased angle of the elbows.

Case Study

Mrs I B came to the prepregnancy clinic with her fourteen-year-old daughter who suffers from Turner's Syndrome. This is a condition with a missing sex chromosome, and so is labelled XO. Such a Monosomy X occurs in roughly 1 in 2,500 newborn females. Elaine, the daughter, was short, had webbing of the neck and her breast development was less than it should be in a girl of fourteen, for her chest was shield-like and she had widely spaced nipples. She had no pubic hair and had not started to menstruate.

Mrs I B wanted to know about Elaine's future reproductive capacity. After checking Elaine's chromosomes in her white blood cells and confirming the diagnosis of Turner's Syndrome, we had to explain to Mrs I B that

(Case Study cont.)

Elaine might never produce eggs and therefore may never be able to reproduce. There are rare reports of pregnancies in women with Turner's Syndrome, fifty-six pregnancies overall, and these occurred in twenty-three women. Even in this minute series, a quarter ended in spontaneous miscarriage and of those who survived, four had Down's Syndrome.

This was sad news to have to break to Elaine and her mother but, armed with this knowledge, they could face the future more realistically, knowing that Elaine's egg reserve was greatly depleted and potential fertility almost nil.

These extra sex chromosomes are produced in the same way as described in Down's Syndrome with its Trisomy 21; there has not been a proper division of the chromosomes in the gametes just before the sperm or the egg was made.

Single Gene Disorders

The genes of a chromosome cannot be seen, even with an electron microscope, but their presence can be calculated from an analysis of the sequence of amino acids. There is no precise size to a gene; they vary from fifty to 2,000,000 nucleic acid sequences. A gene is that part of a chromosome which acts as a functional entity, producing the same characters in all the cells which it enters. If the gene gets the sequence wrong, the malwritten code goes to all cells in the body and will be transmitted by the sperm or egg into other individuals.

A single gene disorder can be either dominant or recessive; if dominant, it can cause the abnormal condition in any individual in which the gene occurs, irrespective of the partner gene. A recessive gene will only cause a clinical problem if the partner's matching gene in the chromosome also has that recessive characteristic. If they both have the condition, then the new individual will show symptoms and signs of the disorder. If only half the chromosomes contain the gene with a recessive code, the bearer will be normal but could be a carrier for that condition, for half his gametes will also bear the recessive gene. Sometimes the condition will not appear in childhood, so that the individual may remain without any signs of the disease until adult. Such a person may not know if they have inherited the condition and could actually be having a family before the clinical signs of the abnormal dominant gene appear. Hence, in genetic counselling at a prepregnancy clinic, it is important to consider the pattern of inheritance through several generations of the family. In addition, the severity of the condition can vary enormously. Although the gene may be present, the amount of influence on the person can be hard to predict.

AUTOSOMAL DOMINANT DISORDERS

Examples are: achondroplasia; adult polycystic kidney disease; some cases of Alzheimer's Disease; Huntington's Chorea; neurofibromatosis; polyps of the colon; and tuberous sclerosis. If there is a family history of any of these conditions on either side, the couple would do well to seek genetic counselling where the risks can be worked out by examination of the full family tree. Before going for prepregnancy care, it would be wise to be prepared with information about members of both families who have suffered any disorder. Some conditions are so severe that they cause babies to die in the uterus or immediately after birth; it requires much tact and detective ability to find out the full story when discussing this aspect with relatives.

Case Study

Mr and Mrs W V were a happy and endearing couple of achondroplastic dwarfs. Full of bounce, they worked in a circus and led a fulfilling life. Now they were wondering about a future family.

In achondroplasia, the growing ends of the long bones fuse to the shafts too soon in early childhood, so that

(Case Study cont.)

whilst the body and head grow to normal size, the limbs do not. As a consequence, the W Vs were 114 cm (3 ft 9 in) and 109 cm (3 ft 7 in) in height respectively. They wanted to know what their chances were of producing normal children and what problems could occur in childbirth.

Unhappily, after working out their family tree, we had to point out they had a 1 in 4 chance of having a highly affected baby who would probably die in the uterus, a 1 in 2 chance of having an affected child and a 1 in 4 chance of having a normal child who would still be a possible carrier. Thus, two out of three living children would be affected and a fourth would die. This was a bad prognosis, and the two dwarfs left our clinic sadly to think about this. We did not see them again, and I fear that our advice, although truthful and maybe helpful, was not what they had expected or wanted.

AUTOSOMAL RECESSIVE DISORDERS

Examples are: cystic fibrosis; dystrophic dwarfism; phenyl-ketonuria; sickle-cell disease and thalassaemia. Research shows that the last two have a higher chance of appearing in Negro populations.

Autosomal inherited disorders are often severe. If a child has already been affected, there is a variable but high risk of recurrence in a subsequent pregnancy – too high a risk to be taken by many couples; antenatal tests on the amniotic fluid or the fetal cells can only be taken once the next pregnancy has started. The only solution possible at the moment is to make a diagnosis in early pregnancy and then to recommend an abortion of that particular embryo in the hope that on the next occasion, the same thing will not recur. First cousin marriages may increase the risk of autosomal recessive disorders. Those with a family history of a genetic disorder should seek prepregnancy advice.

X-LINKED DISORDERS

Chromosomal problems linked to the X chromosome could in theory occur in either sex, for the man (XY) and the woman (XX) both carry an X chromosome. This is true with the X-linked dominant disorders such as vitamin-D-resistant rickets. However, with X-linked recessive disorders, only men are affected, though the disorder may be carried by healthy women. A female carrier would then transmit the disorder to half of her offspring so that half her sons would be affected while half her daughters would become carriers. X-linked recessive disorders cannot be transmitted by a healthy male.

Many X-linked problems are so severe that the fetus dies in the uterus. This is not always so, and examples range from mild conditions such as colour blindness to severe ones such as Duchenne muscular dystrophy. Haemophilia is in this group, as is the increasingly recognized condition of glucose-6-phosphate dehydrogenase deficiency.

Case Study

Probably the most widespread example of X-linked disorder is colour blindness. Mr and Mrs A L came to see us because they were concerned about this. In his youth, Mr A L had wanted to join the Royal Navy but was found to be colour blind at the medical testing stage and was unable to join up. In consequence, he was concerned about the possible effect on his children.

We pointed out to him that nearly always only males are affected by such X-linked recessive disorders (although his daughters might become carriers) and that, generally speaking, the genes are not passed from father to son.

We were able to advise Mr A L of this and he seemed pleased to think that his son might grow up to join the Royal Navy.

Y-LINKED DISORDERS

A Y-linked gene disorder can obviously only affect males, since only they carry a Y chromosome; transmission is directly from father to son. This leads to clinically insignificant abnormalities and is probably responsible for conditions of the skin, such as webbing of the toes.

Various single gene disorders occur in about 7 per 1,000 live births. Sometimes there is warning from the past family history. Anyone who has given birth to a child with these conditions or has a family history of them should have genetic advice in the prepregnancy period.

Multifactorial Disorders

Multifactorial disorders occur in some 20 per 1,000 births and the tendency to produce such abnormalities runs in families. There is no identifiable chromosomal or genetic basis using our current measuring methods. There is probably a combination of multiple genetic characteristics affected by an additional environmental factor. Examples are neural tube defects (spina bifida and anencephaly), congenital heart disease and cleft palate.

Anyone who has had a baby with these conditions should consult a prepregnancy clinic before another pregnancy. After a previous episode of this nature, there is a 3% to 5% risk of a repeat problem but, unlike genetic or chromosomal problems, it is possible to reduce the risks. The environmental factor, which acts in combination with the chromosomal one, may be neutralized by a change of lifestyle. It is possible that adding vitamins to diet around the time of conception could reduce the risk of spina bifida after a previous affected birth as described in Chapter 8.

Case Study

Mrs W P came to us because, being an epileptic receiving treatment, she was wondering about possible problems in a future pregnancy. She was worried that the trait would be passed on to her offspring. She did not appreciate the additional factor that the very treatment she was taking for epilepsy might itself have an effect on the unborn child and so the interview turned into one about her familial history with a multifactorial genetic background and a specific one about drugs in pregnancy.

We discussed the possible effects of the drugs she might be taking on the development of the baby and she accepted that valproic acid derivatives have a low chance of association with a neural-tube defect or craniofacial abnormality. She agreed that she would take her anti-epileptic drugs into consideration when she wanted to start a pregnancy and would discuss them with her neurologist and the prepregnancy clinic staff.

This still left the question of genetic propensity because of her epilepsy and the effect on the embryo of the increased risk of fits during the pregnancy itself if drugs were stopped. Because of the familial history of epilepsy, there was a two-fold increase in the risks of abnormalities to the fetus over and above that of any drugs taken; this was stressed. Further, there was a 25% to 40% chance of increased fits during pregnancy, but their effect on the developing embryo was more difficult to quantify.

Mrs W P listened carefully to all this advice and elected to go onto another anti-epileptic drug in the first three months of pregnancy. She had three *grand mal* fits in pregnancy but was delivered normally of a healthy male child weighing 3.7 kg (8 lb 2 oz) who, after two years follow-up, is normal, has remained well, and is epilepsy-free so far.

Disorders with a Partial Genetic Component

Many diseases run more frequently in families but no true chromosomal or genetic component can be calculated. These include diabetes and epilepsy which have strong family tendencies and are discussed in Chapter 6.

Case Study

Mrs V V was very worried about the chances of her child developing a similar problem to the one she had had. As a baby, Mrs V V had had a narrowing of the muscular valve leading from the stomach (pyloric stenosis) and had required an operation when she was two weeks old.

It had to be explained that the risks of pyloric stenosis depend on multifactorial and inherited factors, so that as well as the risk of the genes being passed across, a number of other factors (such as the number of affected people in the family) could alter the risks of having this condition. In Mrs V V's case, she was the only one of her family for three generations with pyloric stenosis and her husband's family was clear. If a woman has this condition, there is a much greater risk of her passing it on to the next generation; if a man has it, the risk is less. Independently, there is a greater background risk if the child is male rather than female.

It took time to explain these perfectly logical but apparently conflicting factors, and Mrs V V came back again with her husband. The recurrent risk for a boy child in her particular case was about 20% but for a girl child only about 4%.

Mrs V V decided to take these risks and at the time of going to press is still pregnant. An ultrasound of the boy baby in the uterus does not indicate any obvious obstruction at the exit from the stomach.

Heart attacks may have a familial tendency; the narrowing of the coronary arteries of the heart is due partly to the laying down of fat in the walls of the blood vessels. This is mostly an ageing process but may well be affected by the contents of our diet. One variety of early heart disease occurs when there is a familial condition of raised cholesterol levels in the blood, an autosomal dominant trait. This is an unusual condition but a very obvious example of hereditary factors in heart disease. The risk to the closest relatives, especially brothers and sons, of somebody who has had a heart attack before the age of sixty-five is about six times that of the background population.

Certain benign tumours of the nerves (neurofibromata) have a strong familial tendency. These are associated with an autosomal dominant condition. There is an increased risk of cancer of the large bowel among those who have had colonic polyps and here again, an autosomal dominant condition may be involved. In these cases, it is probable that a chemical carcinogen is the final trigger responsible for the stimulation of the actual condition in the cells but the risk is increased by these gene changes.

If there is a family history of any of these conditions the couple would do well to consult their family doctor who can check the likelihood of a genetic component. Subsequent referral to a prepregnancy genetic clinic can help sort out the details of this.

Calculating the Risk

When a couple with a background of hereditary problems attends a prepregnancy clinic, the risk of developing or transmitting a disorder is assessed. If there is a gene disorder, then by taking a history and obtaining details of the rest of the family, a pedigree can be worked out which will give the odds in many cases. For instance, in the autosomal dominant disorders there is a variable chance, up to 1 in 2, of developing the condition in the offspring of one affected parent; very rarely both parents have that condition, and the risk rises to 75%. In the autosomal recessive disorders however, whilst members of the family may be gene carriers, the actual risks are much lower. The chance of a healthy sibling having affected children is low but rises if there is a marriage between blood relatives.

If both parents are affected by a recessive condition, the risk to the offspring depends upon the exact form of the condition and all risks need to be individually calculated. In some cases, the recessive condition may be expected in all the children, in others only some. The X-linked recessive disorders provide complex calculations to the risk and a special genetic centre is usually required to work this out.

Such matters are complex; couples deserve the best advice they can get and should ask their family doctor who will know of the nearest prepregnancy genetic clinic.

Methods of Testing

If a previous baby has been born with an abnormality or there has been a miscarriage, chromosomes from the fetus may have been examined. Scientists can use the skin cells or the white cells of the blood; the latter give quicker results. White cells in the parents' blood can be taken by a simple blood sample from the mother and father and these can be submitted to chromosomal testing.

The method of chromosomal testing is very similar in all parts of the world. After the blood sample is taken, the red cells which predominate greatly in blood are removed by centrifuging; the white cells are removed to be cultured in a special medium under sterile conditions at body temperature for three days. The cells grow and a drug, colchicine, is added to the culture medium to stop any further cell division at the phase when the chromosomes are most dense and clearly defined. The membrane around the nucleus in the cell is dispersed by making it burst so that the chromosomes are spread. These are examined by microscope and the chromosomes from individual, dispersed nuclei are photographed. Enlargements are made so that the chromosomes can be cut out with scissors from the photograph and arranged in pairs to produce a map or karyotype. This is examined carefully for missing chromosomes, additional ones (e.g., Trisomy 21), or fragments joined on to the wrong place (dysjunction). The photographic identification of chromosomes is a very skilled and lengthy process taking several hours. Identification has been aided by fluorescent stains. In research laboratories radiometric methods are used; the cell cultures are exposed to radioactive isotopes which show up the banding pattern of the chromosomes.

To detect chromosomal problems from the baby in the uterus, some fetal cells must first be obtained. For the last thirty years amniocentesis has been used. This is an out-patient procedure, usually performed with local anaesthetic under ultrasound control. Using a syringe and fine needle, fluid from around the fetus is removed; it is then centrifuged to spin down the cells floating in it. These cells come mostly from fetal skin, and to a lesser extent from the lung or bladder lining. They contain the same genetic code as all other fetal cells so, after separation, the cells are cultured under similar conditions to the white cells mentioned already; skin cells, however, are much slower growing than blood cells. Since there are usually not enough skin cells shed into the amniotic fluid until the fetus is about sixteen weeks old, amniocentesis can normally only take place after this time. Because the skin cells are so slow growing, three weeks are required for culture – at least twenty-one days must go by before a result can be obtained. Thus, if the amniocentesis is taken at sixteen weeks, the results will not be available until nineteen weeks' gestation. This is very late in pregnancy for any termination to take place, should the parents request one.

Because it is an invasive procedure, amniocentesis has a small risk of about 1 in 100 to 200 of inducing a miscarriage. This is lessened if done under ultrasound guidance and by an experienced obstetrician.

Case Study

Mrs W W was thirty-eight years old when she first became pregnant and asked at the booking clinic about an amniocentesis. The procedure was explained to her, the doctor concerned being cautious and explaining the 0.5% risk of amniocentesis inducing a miscarriage or being associated with a preterm labour. Mrs W W listened carefully and still decided to have an amniocentesis.

The procedure was performed under ultrasound guidance at sixteen weeks. Ten ml (0.4 fl oz) of clear amniotic fluid were withdrawn and sent to the laboratory. After the amniocentesis, Mrs W W rested in hospital for half a day and then returned home to rest. Unfortunately the following day the uterus started to contract and within half an hour she had ruptured her membranes and clear fluid started coming down the vagina. She returned immediately to the hospital but on examination, the neck of the womb was about 5 cm (2 in) open; a miscarriage followed some five hours later.

This was an unfortunate but known risk of the procedure. Even in retrospect, Mrs W W felt she had taken the right step, for she could not have brought up a child with a chromosomal abnormality. The sad postscript was that three weeks later the result of the tests on the cells removed at the amniocentesis showed a normal chromosomal pattern.

An earlier sampling of the fetal cells can be made by chorionic villus sampling. The definitive placenta is not formed properly until about twelve weeks. Before this time there is excess tissue available. Cells are taken from just off the edge of the growing placenta; they contain chromosomal material identical with the rest of the embryo cells.

This is also an outpatient procedure which is usually performed before the eleventh week of pregnancy. A fine, hollow needle is introduced via the vagina and through the cervix to the edge of the forming placenta; alternatively it can take place under local anaesthetic through the abdominal wall and the muscle of the uterus. In either case, simultaneous ultrasound navigation ensures that the needle arrives in the right place. A small sample of the chorionic tissue is removed by suction for culture. Since there are many active cells and they grow swiftly on culture, a result can be obtained within a week. If a termination of pregnancy has to be recommended, this can be performed at eleven to twelve weeks, a less traumatic procedure than a later operation.

At present, chorionic villus sampling has a slightly higher risk than amniocentesis of being associated with a miscarriage, in the region of 2% to 4% (compared with 0.5% for amniocentesis). However, this does not automatically mean that chorionic villus sampling is four to eight times as dangerous as amniocentesis for the fetus. It must be remembered that at this earlier stage of pregnancy (ten or eleven weeks) there is a much greater chance of spontaneous abortion anyway. At present these methods can be used for DNA diagnoses of cystic fibrosis and muscular dystrophy at most regional genetic centres in the United Kingdon.

Case Study

Mrs D de Q was thirty-seven years old when she became pregnant. She had heard about chorionic villus sampling and came early to the hospital requesting that this be done on the grounds of her age, for she did not want to have a baby with a chromosomal abnormality. She was counselled carefully about the possible problems arising from chorionic villus biopsy. It was explained that although the procedure was carried out early (ten to eleven weeks) and the results came back quickly (in two days), at present there was a 2% to 4% chance of the pregnancy miscarrying afterwards. Mrs D de Q was

(Case Study cont.)

very upset about this and felt that doctors should not be offering a procedure with a high miscarriage rate. It was explained that all procedures have complication rates which are usually high when first introduced but are reduced when the procedure has been performed many more times.

After some discussion, Mrs D de Q asked if there was any other way that the fetus could be tested and we explained that amniocentesis could be performed at about sixteen weeks (with results at about nineteen weeks) and that this had a 0.5% risk. Mrs D de Q immediately brightened and said she would like that; she felt that the risks of the second procedure were so small compared with the first that we ought to recommend it to all women.

The amniocentesis was performed. The results were normal and Mrs D de Q had a healthy baby some months later.

A newer technique, cordocentesis, requires a sample of the fetal blood to be taken directly from the umbilical cord, using a needle under ultrasound control. This is a research technique carried out in special cases only in a few hospitals after eighteen weeks of pregnancy. It allows fetal white blood cells to be obtained and consequently gives quick results on chromosomal abnormalities. This is a new technique and is not yet fully evaluated. In addition to the chromosomal studies however, cordocentesis will allow other investigations into the fetus, including acquired infections, abnormality of the haemoglobin molecule, Rhesus* problems, metabolic congenital abnormalities and an assessment of fetal oxygenation.

Prepregnancy Genetic Counselling
The ideal time for genetic enquiries and for counselling to be given is before the next pregnancy, thus preventing birth

defects rather than detecting them in pregnancy and offering abortion. The couple can consider the risks of the problem and then act accordingly (see Chapter 1). When a couple attends a genetic prepregnancy clinic, they should be prepared for a long interview with much detailed discussion of the whole family history. It may be that questions are asked which need further answers and the couple will have to go away and examine their own family history and return for a second session. As mentioned previously, details will be required about the whole family including information about miscarriages and those who are deceased.

A second source of information is the woman's past obstetrical history. This is a guide to what may happen on another occasion and so any previous miscarriages, babies born with abnormalities or who died, must be discussed. This reopens old wounds but is necessary in order to give a full set of risks for the next pregnancy. Hospital notes may be required and photographs or X-rays taken at the time of the previous pregnancy are extremely helpful. In some cases, autopsies will have been performed or tissue removed for examination. All this will make the discussion more useful to a couple deciding on future pregnancies.

Case Study

Mrs P S came to the prepregnancy clinic and told us the very sad history of her past attempts to have a child. She was thirty-six and had had five pregnancies with no live births. The first occurred when she was twenty-three and she had had a termination at eight weeks, for she was not married and did not know the man concerned very well. She was well afterwards and proceeded to marry in the late 1970s, becoming pregnant in 1980. Unfortunately this ended in a spontaneous miscarriage at twenty-four weeks. There was no obvious cause. This was followed by spontaneous miscarriages at twenty, twenty and eighteen

(Case Study cont.)

weeks respectively at about two-year intervals. She des-
paired and gave up the idea of having a family but,
having heard about prepregnancy counselling, decided
to see what the odds were and so came to discuss them
with us.

We went through her history, gathering as much detail
of each pregnancy as Mrs P S could remember. She
remembered well, for these sad events had impressed
themselves indelibly on her memory. A physical examination of the pelvis revealed no obvious abnormality,
although the neck of the womb did seem a little wide. We
did an X-ray study of the uterus and found the cervix to
be incompetent, for the internal sphincter was open and
would have allowed a funnelling of the membranes into
the cervical canal. In consequence, we recommended
that Mrs P S have a cervical suture early in the next
pregnancy to close up the neck of the womb.

This was agreed and was carried out when she became
pregnant; the pregnancy continued to thirty-eight weeks
when the suture was removed and Mrs P S went into
labour the following day. She had a 2.9 kg (6 lb 8 oz)
baby and was ecstatic, attributing her success to the
prepregnancy clinic's advice.

The effects of diseases in the mother and father also need
to be assessed; these are discussed in detail in Chapter 6.

The Future
Undoubtedly the methods of fetal diagnosis will improve in
the next decade. At present they do not lead to a cure – only
the possibility of detecting the condition after it is formed; the
couple may then elect to continue, aware of the problem, or
they may request a termination of the pregnancy. The likelihood
of actually changing defective parts of chromosomes in early

pregnancy, and thus preventing genetic abnormalities, is now on the horizon. Everybody is watching this onset of genetic engineering with varying degrees of apprehension.

However, like any other branch of science, it can be controlled and no one need be concerned that a race of monsters is likely to be let loose by mad scientists. Instead the advantages of the use of recombinant DNA technology will be disciplined and used to help couples who previously had a very poor chance of producing a normal baby. The details can be obtained from many good books, readily understood by those with an O level knowledge of biology. One of the best is Alan Emery's volume on *The Elements of Medical Genetics*; it contains an excellent chapter on recombinant DNA and genetic engineering which is simply laid out and easily understood.

Essentially, the site on the chromosome must first be identified by radioisotope*-labelled fragments of a DNA probe being placed alongside the suspect areas of the chromosome and showing, by their mismatch in the order of a few molecules, that there is a fault in the DNA molecular ladder. The defective fragment of DNA can be removed with a short extra length of sequences of bases and amino acids at each end. (A gene is a functional unit of the chromosome and is not of a fixed length.) The fragment could be removed mechanically but it is best removed by restriction enzymes which disconnect the DNA at certain sequence-specific sites, where the pattern of bases is recognized by the enzyme.

There are over 300 restriction enzymes, and by choosing combinations, a desired length of DNA can be unzipped from the chromosome. This may then be put alongside a similar normal sequence of DNA from another cell (the easiest source of spare chromosomes is bacteria, from which segments of DNA can be removed.) Having been checked alongside the human DNA, the donor section is introduced into the cell and division takes place so that the new healthy DNA segment is incorporated with the matching segment of original DNA. Thus the foreign fragment is now part of the chromosome and a healthy chain has been produced. This is grown and cultured to produce a series of clones or equal biological segments of DNA. The correctness of the sequence of bases and amino acids can be checked by radioactive gene-specific probes.

This is about as far as most scientists have come at the moment. To go further would mean that having made the relevant DNA segment, this gene section of the chromosome, complete with its control sequences at either end, would be reintroduced into the isolated host cells and into the human chromosomes. At present this has not been achieved with any certainty, though some research workers do report results in other species.

Recombinant DNA work is useful already: it can pick on a gene site precisely and, with radioisotope precision, spot the actual point on any given chromosome where the faulty genetic factor was carried. Many of these faults have been localized and the site of a large number of genetic potential sites on several of the chromosomes has now been mapped. This allows diagnostic precision to be improved when chorionic villus tissue is removed and a more precise diagnosis can be made to help the couple. Good examples of this are in cystic fibrosis and certain haemoglobin abnormalities such as some thalassaemias. It is not yet possible to provide treatment by replacing the affected gene but this will probably happen in the near future.

Such research and its application must be carefully considered and its organization guarded. In Britain, the government central committee, the Genetic Manipulation Advisory Group (GMAG), lays down very thorough guidelines for research. Members of the group inspect laboratories doing this work and other government organizations watch this area carefully. When scientific advances are made in this field, they will be of help to many couples who at the moment can only produce abnormal babies.

Conclusions

Characteristics are carried from one cell to another by means of coded messages in the chromosomes. Each position of every chromosome is carefully loaded with a genetic plan for the future cells. Abnormalities in chromosomes can lead to disorders of development. All chromosomes exist in pairs, one coming from each parent. Abnormalities may be carried on the ordinary chromosomes or on the sex chromosomes. If the latter, then the condition will only occur in children of the appropriate sex.

Many of these abnormalities can be tested for in early pregnancy by examination of a small number of fetal cells. This might be very early on in pregnancy, at nine to eleven weeks, by chorionic villus sampling, or by means of amniocentesis later in pregnancy at sixteen to eighteen weeks. In some medical centres the DNA may also be examined in detail, looking at the precise sites on chromosomes where faults have occurred, thus diagnosing exactly what condition will result.

FIVE

Inbuilt Biological Factors

Let her shun disquietness of mind, anger, vexing and grief: for if a woman did but see her own face in a glass when she is in such passions, she would hire a man to throw stones at it.

Culpeper

When a couple consults a doctor at a prepregnancy clinic, he or she is faced with certain fixed biological features in that couple which have been laid down long before they arrived at the clinic. These include biological and social aspects of the couple's life, their past health, as well as, in certain cases, what happened in previous pregnancies. All these factors can indicate the risks of problems in the next pregnancy and the hazards must be assessed by the pregnancy counsellor; where events have taken place which cannot be altered, the related risks must be fully discussed with the couple so as to allow them to make an informed choice.

Age

The mother's age has a pronounced effect on the outcome of pregnancy, that of the father has less. For a few years after the start of menstruation, most of the cycles are not associated with egg-making. From sixteen to twenty years, eggs are made in about two-thirds of cycles, but from then to about the age of thirty-five, most cycles in the majority of women include ovulation. Once the woman is over forty, the proportion of cycles without an egg rises again until the menopause, by which time all the primordial eggs have been used up from the ovaries. Hence, in the middle part of reproductive life, when intercourse is more frequent, there is a greater likelihood of eggs being produced and the woman becoming pregnant. In the later phase, after thirty-five, intercourse is less frequent and, combined with irregular ovulation, leads to a lower fertility rate characteristic of this decade.

In Chapter 2, we saw how a woman is born with all the primordial (potential) eggs she is going to use. Hence, as a woman ages, these potential eggs are also ageing. There is therefore an increased risk of abnormalities for they have been exposed longer to various influences such as radiation, and so may undergo genetic changes. The most common of these is that the chromosome on position 21 does not divide equally when the helix is split to make the primary egg. In consequence, there are two chromosomes in position 21 instead of one. When that egg proceeds to be fertilized, a third chromosome comes from the sperm and so the condition of Trisomy 21* or Down's Syndrome* starts immediately at the moment of fertilization. The incidence of this condition is very low until the age of thirty-five, increases slightly from then to forty, and is especially high after that time, leading to a risk level of about 1 in 100 at forty, and 5 in 100 by the age of forty-five. Other variations found more frequently in the older woman are multiple pregnancies and the absence of one of the pair of umbilical arteries which may be associated with abnormalities in the fetus.

As well as these chromosomal considerations, a woman past the age of thirty-five must be reminded that she has a higher incidence of the degenerative diseases of life. These usually come on in the forties and fifties but can start earlier, so that a woman of thirty-five years or above has a greater risk than her younger sister of raised blood pressure or diabetes. These can be checked for and their worst side effects guarded against, but they are there.

With increasing maternal age comes a lack of flexibility of the ligaments and the muscles. Pregnancy becomes a greater burden than it would be in the younger woman and increased rest will be needed. Particularly at risk are the ligaments of the back, for with the large mass in the growing abdomen, the back arches like that of the base drummer in a marching band. The drummer puts his drum down occasionally for a rest but the woman cannot put down her growing baby. With the added problem of increased progesterone levels causing softening of the ligaments (as discussed in Chapter 2), a woman is more likely to get small tears and permanent stretches in these ligaments, so producing a back problem. This occurs particularly in women with long backs (i.e., a woman with a long body size) and should be guarded against carefully by watching for over-activity in pregnancy and avoiding it if possible.

For these reasons, any woman seen at the prepregnancy clinic in the older reproductive age should be advised that when she becomes pregnant, she may have to adjust her lifestyle. If forewarned, arrangements can often be made at the same time as planning for the pregnancy. If that advice only comes once the pregnancy has started, it is often too late and the woman will be disappointed and resentful. There is a sliding scale of probable complications which worsen after the age of thirty-five and these should be freely discussed at the prepregnancy clinic. Over this age a woman needs to watch pregnancy more carefully and plan ahead to circumvent the changes in pregnancy.

Previous Pregnancies

The effects of increasing family size on women must be similar to those for age, for they march together. However, there are some aspects associated with further pregnancies which in most societies do not appear until three or four children have been born. After this, there is an increased laxity of the muscle wall of the uterus which can lead to the fetus not fitting in the best position – a longitudinal lie – but lying transversely across the uterus. Further, the neck of the womb might be lax and this would allow the membranes around the baby to bulge down; in very early labour they may rupture, allowing a gush of amniotic fluid to escape, carrying with it the umbilical cord. This would be exceedingly dangerous, for it would mean the communicating lines between mother and baby would be interrupted. In addition, after delivery of the baby, the uterus might not contract on the placenta and placental bed as it should and so extra bleeding could occur and a postpartum haemorrhage take place. Such risks should be considered when discussing the effects of increased family size.

In the United Kingdon, the mean family size is now about 2.1 – many women do not have more children after the second and so these problems of increased parity do not exist. However, 5% of women in the United Kingdom, some of whom come from other countries, still have large families and they are seen at the prepregnancy clinics of this country. If you already have a large family, it is wise to discuss possible problems at a prepregnancy clinic and to take this opportunity to learn what effect the next pregnancy may have on you and on your existing family, for there may be restrictions placed upon your activity in the forthcoming pregnancy which need long-term planning.

Past Reproductive Experience

Many women attending the prepregnancy clinic have had a pregnancy before which has finished unhappily. There may have been a spontaneous miscarriage in early pregnancy or although pregnancy continued there were problems with delivery. Theoretically, the best time to discuss these matters would have been just after the miscarriage or delivery. Then the doctor who actually dealt with the woman would have had all the notes available and would have been able to discuss the implications of various events. However, people often wish to get away from sad episodes and the woman may have left the hospital swiftly after a miscarriage and not returned for the proffered follow-up visit. Similarly, after delivery she may have wished to go home and return to her own ambience, and she may not even have gone for the postnatal visit. Even if the woman has kept these appointments, she may have been seen by a junior doctor who was not acquainted with her case, or a General

Practitioner who was sent only a short summary of events. If something which worries the woman or her partner occurs in pregnancy or labour, the wisest thing is to ask to speak to the senior obstetrician fairly soon. In the United Kingdom, a consultant, if asked, will always make himself or herself readily available and discuss the matter very soon after the event.

Case Study

Mrs E K was very worried about future pregnancies. She already had three children and with each there had been a problem.

In the first pregnancy, she had had high blood pressure. Mrs E K was admitted to hospital and had to be induced at thirty-five weeks. Labour did not proceed well and she was delivered by forceps after fetal distress. The baby weighed only 1.8 kg (4 lb) and had a stormy time in the neonatal unit but eventually did well.

In her second pregnancy, Mrs E K was watched very carefully in the outpatient clinic but did not have raised blood pressure. However, she went into spontaneous labour at thirty-four weeks and produced a 1.4 kg (3 lb 2 oz) baby who was remarkably resilient and required only a minimum of help in the Special Care Baby Unit.

Two years ago, Mrs E K again became pregnant and again escaped any raised blood pressure but went into labour at thirty-six weeks, producing on this occasion a larger child, 2.2 kg (4 lb 8 oz), who required little attention. Sadly, however, this child died of sudden infant death syndrome (cot death) at five months and Mrs E K felt that her reproductive future was doomed.

We went into each of these cases carefully with her. The records of two were in our own hospital notes whilst the third was obtained easily, for it was at a hospital nearby. With all these records, we were able to discuss Mrs E K's past pregnancies fully at a second interview.

Problems could be summarized as follows:

1 *The raised blood pressure* had occurred in the first pregnancy but not in the two subsequent ones. The chances of this happening again were fairly low.

2 *The fetal distress* only occurred in the first pregnancy and therefore the chances of its recurrence were no greater than background.

3 *The cot death* was after the most recent pregnancy and so the chances of its happening again might be slightly increased. This was discussed in detail with Mrs E K.

4 *The early labour* was most likely to be a recurrent problem but we were able to point out to Mrs E K that in the last two cases, the babies had not been greatly affected initially. However, one had suffered cot death and there was a slight association between Sudden Infant Death Syndrome and preterm deliveries. This we discussed fully.

After a long interview, Mr and Mrs E K were grateful for this analysis of their past obstetrical history and felt they could go into another pregnancy more happily and with a greater knowledge of the odds. This is a good example of the non-specific, general help that a prepregnancy clinic can offer.

We heard a year later that Mrs E K had had another baby who was born at thirty-five weeks, weighing 2 kg (4 lb 5 oz). When she wrote to us the baby was six months old and doing well.

This advice is the ideal; unfortunately some women do not see a senior doctor after a problem birth and so at the prepregnancy clinic we see many women who had a problem in the previous pregnancy and fear a recurrence the next time.

Past Miscarriages

Spontaneous miscarriage is a common event. Many used to think that there was a steeply rising risk of recurrence as the number of miscarriages increased. This is not true. After one miscarriage, there is a doubling of the risk and after two consecutive miscarriages, the odds may go up so that about one-third of future pregnancies may miscarry. That still leaves two-thirds of pregnancies likely to continue to the delivery of a normal baby. What is more, the risks do not increase greatly after this but reach a plateau; so women need not feel, because they have had three, four or even five miscarriages, that they have increased the risk every time. It would seem that the risk of repeated miscarriage relates not so much to the number of previous miscarriages but to the closeness of any previous miscarriage in the pregnancy order. The prepregnancy counsellor can advise the woman about any specific reasons for miscarriage which may be disguised by the general figures just given, but the chances of producing a live, normal baby are probably still much greater than 1 in 2. Such news is encouraging to many women who persevere and are happily rewarded.

These odds can be discussed in detail with the prepregnancy counsellor who will give specific advice. He or she will probably also discuss the possibility of structural abnormalities of the uterus such as a septum or partition down the middle of the cavity, and may also investigate cervical incompetence. The other major group of causes of spontaneous miscarriages is based on recurring congenital abnormalities of the embryo so severe that the embryo cannot even survive in the uterus. Development is therefore halted and the embryo is absorbed or miscarries. Here the advice of a genetic clinic may be sought (see Chapter 4).

Other Biological Factors

Low Birth Weight

The risks of death and illness rise greatly the more immature the baby is at birth; a baby with a very low birth weight has greatly reduced chances of survival. Low birth weight might follow too early a delivery or retardation of fetal growth inside the uterus. These two conditions sometimes exist together, but the prepregnancy counsellor will try to distinguish between the two and help the couple work out the risks of producing a baby that is too small in further pregnancy.

PRETERM LABOUR

Causes of a preterm delivery are not always known. Low-grade infection of the upper vagina and uterus may be associated with early membrane rupture. In other cases, the membranes spontaneously rupture prematurely and this is swiftly followed by labour. The risks of this need to be discussed with the prepregnancy counsellor so that advice may be given. This may involve planned admission to hospital for some time well before the baby is due. If this has happened before, the timing of admission will relate to what occurred previously. When this is discussed and agreed before pregnancy starts, it is often much easier to implement.

If the obstetrician decides that the baby would be safer outside the uterus than in he or she would either induce labour or perform an elective Caesarean section. This might be done when the mother has raised blood pressure, is bleeding from the vagina or the baby is not growing in the uterus. The chances of all such problems recurring should be discussed with the prepregnancy clinic counsellor who will give appropriate odds in each individual case.

Sometimes, there is a multiple pregnancy; these often finish early. The normal length of gestation in the woman with a single baby is forty weeks, but the average pregnancy with twins would be thirty-seven weeks and triplets thirty-two weeks. Multiple pregnancies are more common after ovulation has been induced, so women who are undergoing treatment of this nature should consult a prepregnancy clinic. The chances of having twins are much greater after gonadotrophin* stimulation of the ovaries than with clomiphene* treatment; those who have previously had a spontaneous multiple pregnancy have a slightly increased chance of its happening again. Such women would be advised to attend the prepregnancy clinic early in the next pregnancy so that the diagnosis could be made with ultrasound by sixteen weeks and then plans laid for the pregnancy. Some obstetricians may advise rest in hospital for longer than in the previous pregnancy.

In about half the cases of previous preterm delivery, no specific cause can be identified and only general advice can be offered. At the prepregnancy clinic, the increased risk of another preterm pregnancy will be emphasized whatever the cause; associated factors should be borne in mind. The best course of action is for the woman to attend her antenatal clinic early in a subsequent pregnancy so that progress can be properly monitored. It may be wise to consider the use of uterine relaxant drugs in the middle of pregnancy, or if the cervix is incompetent, further pregnancies may be at increased risk of premature ending. A little dilatation in the opening of the neck of the womb could allow the membranes around the growing baby to bulge down and so rupture early, leading to a miscarriage or a preterm labour. Some obstetricians would advise that this be guarded against by putting in a purse-string stitch around the cervix in the next pregnancy. This would be inserted under general anaesthetic high up in the cervix, constricting the canal to prevent membrane bulge. This treatment is successful for some women and the prepregnancy clinic will advise whether or not it would be suitable for a particular individual.

It is possible that the woman's lifestyle will have to be altered; work done outside the home may have to be curtailed and that in the home reduced in the middle weeks of pregnancy. Sexual intercourse can be a stimulant to preterm labour and so may have to be avoided. All such factors should be discussed in more detail at the prepregnancy clinic and plans made well before the birth.

RETARDED GROWTH IN THE UTERUS

Because of a diminished blood supply to the placental bed, some babies do not grow at a normal rate inside the uterus. This can be associated with raised blood pressure although it is not always so. Reduced blood flow results not only in a baby who has a low birth weight but may also lead to longer-term mental or even physical handicap. If this has happened in a previous pregnancy, the couple would do well to seek prepregnancy advice before embarking on another baby. The prepregnancy counsellor will go into these matters with them and try to locate a cause. As already indicated, the actual reason is a reduction in placental bed blood flow but the background for this might not be immediately apparent. For instance, smoking may affect the placental bed blood flow as can excess alcohol intake. Hence, any woman with a previous history of a small-for-dates baby would be well advised to stop or reduce smoking and alcohol intake well before pregnancy.

Research in this subject is advancing. In certain obstetrical hospitals placental bed blood flow can be assessed in a non-invasive fashion by reflecting sound waves from the blood vessels in the placental bed. Ultrasound waves are beamed onto the blood vessels and, when reflected back, give a measure of the speed of the wave of blood through the uterine arteries. This can be estimated by very sensitive equipment and, from it, some estimate of the blood flow through the placental bed arteries can be obtained. Further, the blood flow through the umbilical vessels can also be measured and this shows the ability of the fetus to obtain nutrients and oxygen from the placenta in later pregnancy.

This is not a painful procedure and uses no harmful rays so that it has no effect on the growing child. If offered, it would be wise to use this test; a woman who has had a previous baby with intrauterine growth retardation may do well to consider booking into a hospital that offers such tests. Further, she will be seen more frequently in the antenatal clinic and may be admitted during pregnancy. Such extra surveillance during pregnancy must be accepted if pregnancy is to produce its best result. Hence a change of activities may have to be planned.

Death rates amongst babies under 1 kg (2 lb 3 oz) birth weight are diminishing rapidly thanks to the proper use of obstetrical preventive care and neonatal intensive-care units. There are one or two intensive-care units in every region of the United Kingdom and the couple should enquire about these before pregnancy. Indeed, the woman may be wise to book her delivery in a hospital where one of these units is available, in order to give her next child the best chance. However, some babies born after a previous child with intrauterine growth retardation are perfectly normal and can be looked after by the paediatric facilities in a district hospital near the woman's home. Advice will depend on each individual case and many prepregnancy counsellors would not be dogmatic at this stage but would suggest a policy of awaiting events and transferring the booking if the need arises in the next pregnancy.

Raised Blood Pressure

About one in ten women suffer from pre-eclampsia or raised blood pressure in their first pregnancy. If there are no underlying grounds for raised blood pressure, the risks of this happening in the second and subsequent pregnancies are greatly reduced. Hence, it is reasonable to reassure couples that severe pre-eclampsia is less likely to recur and that the chances of its not recurring are better in a subsequent pregnancy. A small number of women, however, show a recurrent pattern and they should be watched very carefully to rule out any unsuspected causes of blood pressure elevation from the kidney or the adrenal glands. If a woman has previously had raised blood pressure, she should attend for antenatal care early next time in order that the blood pressure can be checked at an early stage.

A slightly different situation arises in a woman who has changed her partner since the last pregnancy. With a new partner, there is a slight increase in the odds that there will be recurrent raised blood pressure in pregnancy; this is probably due to changed immunological patterns introduced by the new partner. The risk can be discussed at the prepregnancy clinic where the woman would learn of the possible lines of treatment that may follow any raised blood pressure in a subsequent pregnancy.

Rhesus Problems

The Rhesus* problem is diminishing rapidly in the United Kingdom, following the prophylactic programme of immunization given to most Rhesus negative women after delivery. Only a small number develop anti-D Rhesus antibodies in pregnancy now, and most of these occur following a mismatched blood transfusion or failure to obtain anti-D immunization in a previous pregnancy. Any Rhesus negative woman who has had a previous Rhesus positive baby should have been given advice and offered inoculation after the last delivery. If she was not inoculated, she should attend a prepregnancy counselling session before thinking of another pregnancy. Here details will be taken of her past pregnancies and her partner's Rhesus state. This may involve blood tests for her partner which might show that he is producing all his sperm with a Rhesus positive feature so that the next baby is bound to be Rhesus positive. If only half the sperm are Rhesus positive then there is a 1 in 2 chance the next child will be Rhesus negative. The severity of Rhesus disease in a previous pregnancy is very important in calculating the prognosis and details may have to be obtained from other hospitals if the woman has moved home meanwhile.

Case Study

Mrs Y H was Rhesus negative. She had known this from her first delivery fifteen years ago; her husband was Rhesus positive. Their first baby was now aged fourteen and was a normal, noisy adolescent. Two years later, when pregnant again, she was found to have Rhesus antibodies at the booking visit. The level of these had increased by twenty-eight weeks. She was retested at thirty weeks when the level of the antibodies had again risen sharply. In consequence, labour was induced at thirty-one weeks and a 0.9 kg (2 lb) baby was born needing two exchange transfusions for she was very jaundiced and had a low haemoglobin count. However, she survived and she, too, is progressing normally at school.

Mrs Y H had a less happy subsequent obstetrical history, for eight years ago the next child died in the uterus at twenty-six weeks before any treatment could be given. The fourth pregnancy was managed at a special Rhesus centre. Despite the high antibodies, Mrs Y H elected to proceed through the pregnancy and the baby was sustained by intraperitoneal transfusions at twenty-two and twenty-four weeks. Despite this, the baby died in the uterus at twenty-five weeks.

Mrs Y H came to us wondering what her chances were now, for she had remarried. We checked her husband's blood at the prepregnancy clinic; he was Rhesus positive but of the variety that does not produce a Rhesus positive baby every time. We advised Mrs Y H of the treatments that can be had for babies and the chances of their success.

She elected to become pregnant and this time the antibody levels did not change in early pregnancy. We checked the blood of the fetus at twenty weeks and found the child was Rhesus negative, the egg having been fertilized by chance with one of the husband's

Rhesus negative sperms. Hence we could assure Mrs Y H that there would be no problems with this pregnancy. Indeed, she went through to thirty-nine weeks when she had a spontaneous labour, producing a 3.2 kg (7 lb 1 oz) girl who was quite normal.

If a woman has several severely affected babies due to Rhesus disease, then there are specialized treatments that may be appropriate. These include maternal total plasma exchange in pregnancy for which couples must be referred to special centres. Rhesus disease is unusual in the United Kingdom now and so not all hospitals deal with it. However, each region has a Rhesus centre where expert advice can be given; referral may have to be to that hospital for antenatal care and delivery. Such advice is better considered in the prepregnancy time to allow major family decisions to be made.

Late Intrauterine Death

This is a particularly sad form of perinatal loss; any couple who has experienced a late pregnancy death before will naturally be apprehensive during the next pregnancy right up to the end. Sometimes a mature, apparently normal baby, has been progressing well and in the last weeks of pregnancy, his movements have stopped; on checking, the fetal heartbeat is no longer present. After delivery, examination of the baby and placenta may reveal no obvious abnormalities. Such cases are few but when they happen, the couple should discuss events with their obstetrician just after the delivery. If this is not possible, then they should go into events carefully with the prepregnancy counsellor who will have to write to the previous hospital for medical records.

In the next pregnancy, the baby will be monitored carefully. If necessary, arrangements may have to be made for the woman to be admitted to hospital in the last weeks of the next pregnancy. Labour may be induced early to avoid the previous stillbirth zone and in the vast majority of these cases the next baby is perfectly normal. However, since the cause of the previous stillbirth is not known, counsellors have to take a blanket of extra precautions to cover the next pregnancy and this is best planned in the prepregnancy clinic.

Socio-Economic Class

In Great Britain, the population has a wide spread of social characteristics. Education, living habits and diet vary enormously but tend to group together according to lifestyle – usually a combination of what fits in with friends and neighbours, and what people can afford. Few of us live in palaces and few in hovels. Therefore some more subtle means of differentiating social class is required. This is usually done by a classification based upon the occupation of the male partner. This is not intentionally chauvinistic but supplies a better differentiation than using the woman's occupation as studies show that female employment tends to group around the home or posts connected with secretarial work. Hence the partner's post is used for here there is a wider range of gradation than occurs in female activities.

The relationship between the partner's work and socio-economic status gives an approximate indication of the woman's place in society, revealing aspects of her health and upbringing in infancy – nutrition, the childhood diseases she may have had, education, attitudes to medical care and her genetic inheritance. All these factors influence a woman's obstetrical performance. There is a strong correlation between socio-economic grouping and the incidence of many types of obstetrical problems and reduced birth weight of the infant. With the improvements of medicine in relation to childbearing, it is now probable that the socio-economic structure of the population has as great an influence on the variations of outcome for the baby as does the provision of medical care and facilities. A good example of this is personal habits such as cigarette smoking which tend to be related to socio-economic class.

Cutting across the sociobiological processes is the economic handicap of unemployment. In recent years this has increased greatly and its influence on health has been questioned. In the prepregnancy period, it is hard to believe that the involuntary unemployment of the woman or her partner does not have some influence on early pregnancy and the development of the unborn child. However, any such effects may be mixed with other aspects of stress and nutrition. There are few solid research results published yet, although there may be in a decade's time. Until then the relationship between unemployment and prepregnancy health must remain a question mark.

Socio-economic class is an important predictor of a woman's obstetrical performance, but is not one that in itself can be changed. She may be advised of the hazards that she risks and be counselled at the prepregnancy clinic so that she avoids as many as possible. While no woman can resign from her assigned socio-economic class, for she is set in it, she can take advice at the prepregnancy clinic to reduce its worst influences. She could, for example, improve her diet and her approach to exercise and smoking.

Race

Like socio-economic class, race is a marker of a couple's background and may include factors of varying relevance, depending on the part of the world they come from. Over 1,000 years ago in Britain, the Germans and Danes invaded and occupied the centre and south of the islands, pushing the Celts out to the periphery, to the South-West, Wales and the North. These historical events are still reflected today in increased problems of obstetrical outcome found in these areas.

After the Second World War, the West Indians and the Asians represented two big groups of modern immigrants.

Large groups of Asians settled in the West Midlands and London regions whilst other groups of the West African and Caribbean population came to London and the East Midlands. As an example, in the hospital in which the author works in South London, 16% of the women having babies are Afro-Caribbean and 15% come from the sub-continent of India. Hence, the new immigrants make up one-third of our hospital's women having babies. In other parts of the country, such as Scotland, new immigrants are rare.

The differences that racial origin may produce in a woman's reproductive potential relate to the genetics of her natural background; for example, the incidence of thalassaemia and sickle-cell disease is higher in some races. Further, the upbringing of the woman and her partner in their own country may have led to attitudes which differ from those of the indigenous population. The schooling and educational philosophy of their youth may have been different so that they were brought up with differing ideas, or in another faith. This may affect the use of antenatal care or medical services generally, for their attitude may be less receptive. Nutrition in the country of origin may have been very different and this may have affected growth and development in infancy (this is discussed further in Chapter 8). Finally, women may carry diseases endemic in their country of origin; some women have malaria or other tropical diseases which continue to affect them when they arrive in the United Kingdom.

All new immigrants live in a very different environment from that of their early lives. Often a couple will come to the United Kingdom having had a much higher standard of living in their own country. The factors of nutrition in their youth, education in their childhood and genetic and disease background which exist in even the best-integrated groups must be considered at the prepregnancy clinic when a couple attend. The thalassaemias and sickle-cell diseases are obvious examples. In the prepregnancy service run by the author in South London, if the woman comes from the Mediterranean coastal regions, the West Indies or West Africa, she is offered screening tests on her blood for potential thalassaemia and sickle-cell disease.

Such background factors can give rise to anxiety, and any couple concerned about their background should take prepregnancy advice in order to learn the truth about their problems. Often they will have listened to folk lore about reproductive problems which may have been greatly exaggerated; they will generally be reassured by advice given in the prepregnancy clinic as they will learn of the true risks and can then act upon these. This is a most important area of prepregnancy care and all couples who are concerned about their biological background are strongly advised to take advice at a local prepregnancy clinic.

Conclusions

When a couple consults at the prepregnancy clinic, they come with certain fixed biological and social aspects. These cannot be undone and they may have an effect on the future family; hence they must be considered. Although these factors cannot be changed, the odds relating to possible problems can be calculated and the couple better informed.

Amongst the factors to consider are the mother's and father's age, their past health and what has happened in previous pregnancies. The past reproductive experience of a woman bears strikingly on what might happen in future pregnancies; if there have been problems, then they can be prepared for or avoided. Other inbuilt factors in the couple's background are upbringing, education and social habits. Finally certain problems of pregnancy may relate to the mother's and father's country of origin.

Section IV

FACTORS INFLUENCING OUTCOME

SIX

Previous Illness
and Current Treatment

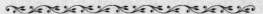

How the . . . body of the parent conduceth to
the life of the child . . . it stirs up natural heat
in them. There is much difference between
a body when natural heat is stirred up, and
when it is not stirred up, as there is between
the earth in winter and summer. When the sun
stirs up natural heat in the elements, the earth
rejoyceth and brings forth its increase. When
the sun departs and by its distance cannot stir
up natural heat, then the earth is dismantled of
the beauty bestoweth upon her and mourns
like the trees in October.

Culpeper

The majority of women who are pregnant are in the sixteen to thirty-five-year age group, a time when most are perfectly healthy. They may have suffered childhood infectious diseases, but the common medical problems in this age group are accidents, producing injuries to limbs, and appendicitis. All these are dealt with at the time of the incident and usually have little effect on pregnancy.

However, a few women suffer from chronic illness and they may be concerned about what is going to happen in pregnancy. They are usually anxious about the effect of the disease itself upon the pregnancy and the unborn child, but should also be conscious of the converse effect which the pregnancy may produce on the advance of the disease. There is much loose thinking which leads to the belief that pregnancy always causes any disease to deteriorate; this is rarely true provided there is proper supervision of the woman throughout the pregnancy and the delivery. Further, the medicines and drugs given for the disease might affect pregnancy and the unborn child more than the disease itself. Many chronic diseases require long-term regimens of drug therapy; these should be carefully surveyed in the prepregnancy clinic in order to see if it is possible to allow the best chance of starting the first few months of pregnancy uninfluenced by these drugs.

In consequence, anyone with a chronic illness should attend a specialist prepregnancy clinic and go into the details of their problem. Specialists are highly skilled; they may not be quite so familiar, however, with the problems that pregnancy can cause in relation to their speciality. Similarly, many obstetricians who are familiar with and skilled in the management of pregnancies may not be *au fait* with the pathological process of a chronic disease. The opinions of the two should come together in the prepregnancy clinic where the obstetrician can consult specialists from other disciplines and consider how pregnancy might worsen the outlook of the disease or vice versa.

Case Study

Mrs B W and her husband came to the prepregnancy clinic. She had ulcerative colitis which had been present for about eight years, and had been treated with steroids and sulphasalazine. She had been told by the gastroenterologist looking after her that she must not contemplate pregnancy for 'it would make the ulcerative colitis worse'.

After full discussion at the prepregnancy clinic, we said we would like to consult the doctor who was looking after the colitis; we wrote to him and explained that ulcerative colitis did not worsen in pregnancy; indeed, a certain proportion of women got better. We pointed out the small but known risks of both steroids and sulphasalazine in producing congenital abnormalities and the very small risks of steroid suppression of the adrenal glands. The gastroenterologist telephoned and we had a useful conversation, deciding that Mrs B W could stop her sulphasalazine for a few months and reduce her steroids. This would give her time to become pregnant and would also remove the risks in the phase of fetal development in early pregnancy. We would see how the ulcerative colitis progressed during the pregnancy and be prepared to restart the sulphasalazine if necessary.

This plan being agreed, Mrs B W and her husband met us again at the prepregnancy clinic and we outlined the suggested management. They accepted this, and Mrs B W is at the moment in late pregnancy; so far her ulcerative colitis has been much better and we have not needed to restart the sulphasalazine.

All prepregnancy care should take place in conjunction with the recommendations of the doctors, both obstetricians and General Practitioners who may be looking after the woman when the pregnancy occurs. Ideally, plans should be made in consultation with the other relevant doctors to save the woman and her partner having to sort out a series of conflicting recommendations made in good faith by different people looking at the same problem from different points of view. This is an important exercise which any woman who has had an established illness should consider; if sought out in good time before pregnancy the experts' advice can help the woman plan her pregnancy. For example, women with certain forms of heart disease may have to be admitted to hospital weeks before delivery. No one likes to be put into this situation, but if the mother-to-be knows that this plan is best for her she can then make arrangements in advance and so limit the disruption to herself, her household and other members of the family. It was for this reason – planning ahead for women with medical problems – that prepregnancy clinics were first started.

The remainder of this chapter will be devoted to short accounts of what a woman may expect from the interaction of pregnancy and her pre-existing disorder. The section may be skipped by the majority of readers who are fortunate enough to have good health, but is included for the few who have certain diseases already. It is hoped they will benefit from learning about possible methods of management that may be adopted in future pregnancies.

Heart Disease

Improved living standards in the Western world have led to a great reduction in rheumatic fever in childhood which in turn has been followed by a reduction in the numbers of young women with rheumatic heart disease. This condition accounts for most of the heart problems in the pregnancy age group. Rheumatic inflammation leads to damage of the heart muscle causing irregularities of the pulse and also to the valves of the heart leading to constrictions and turbulence in the smooth flow of blood. Stenosis or narrowing of the mitral valve is the most common single problem, leading to a damming-back of blood returning to the heart from the lungs. Hence fluid accumulates in the lungs, producing a shortage of breath.

Pregnancy imposes extra stress on the whole body including the heart. On average, a woman increases her blood volume by about 40% in pregnancy; the heart rate increases by about 10%; and the amount of blood pumped out at each beat goes up by 30%. In all, there is a 50% increase in the output of the heart and the work it does. During labour the cardiac work load is increased even further. Each time the uterus contracts it squeezes about 600 ml of blood back into the circulation so that there has to be an increase in cardiac output to cope with this. The pain and anxieties of labour may also affect the blood pressure through the sympathetic nervous system, whilst immediately after delivery the blood squeezed out from the uterus to the general circulation causes another temporary increase in volume. The stability of the blood-circulating systems of the body changes greatly in pregnancy. This could be more than the heart can cope with if it is not functioning at its best capacity. The most common result of this would be that the woman's heart becomes inefficient and so she suffers heart failure with shortage of breath.

An increasing number of women who were born with congenital heart conditions are now leading normal adult lives and some are even becoming pregnant. With the better facilities available for cardiac support, such women now lead more ordinary lives, whereas twenty-five years ago they were severely restricted. Deliveries are also occurring among women who have had heart transplants.

Case Study

Mrs N O knew that she had heart disease. She had had rheumatic fever as a child and was told she had a 'delicate heart'. She was advised not to take part in games and to avoid all exertion. At the age of nineteen she married and came to the prepregnancy clinic because she was frightened about pregnancy.

When we saw Mrs N O and her new husband we discussed the matter fully and started the usual series of investigations. We asked our cardiologist, who shares the care of heart disease in pregnancy, to assess her and he gave Mrs N O an almost clean bill of health; the rheumatic fever had caused a mild narrowing of the mitral valve of the heart but this would probably not have any effect providing pregnancy was watched carefully. Mrs N O accepted the need for extra rest during her pregnancy. She elected to go on working at her desk job in the Civil Service and we concurred.

Pregnancy followed and passed uneventfully. She gave up work at about twenty-eight weeks but at no time was there any deterioration of the heart function. She had a brisk, normal delivery and gave birth to a 3.3 kg (7 lb 4 oz) boy; she and the baby were perfectly well after delivery.

She was pleased she had taken prepregnancy advice and said: 'It eased a lot of anxiety just before pregnancy started and I knew the plans of what might happen during the pregnancy.'

Any woman who knows that she has heart disease should go for prepregnancy advice. The aim would be to assess her heart status as precisely as possible before pregnancy starts; more accurate advice could then be given about the problems that might subsequently arise in pregnancy. The risk of major problems may be so great that a woman might decide not to become pregnant. If there are lesser problems, she may decide to go ahead and accept treatment to minimize those risks. The full assessment of the heart condition would be performed by the prepregnancy counsellor and a cardiologist. Simple, non-invasive tests, such as electrocardiography* and echocardiography* would probably be performed. Using the results from these, the prepregnancy team could advise her of changes that might occur in pregnancy and any strains that these might place on her heart.

The risks of inherited congenital heart lesions will obviously concern the couple seeking prepregnancy advice; this varies with the type of heart disease and needs individual assessment. For women with artificial heart valves, the problems of anticoagulation during pregnancy should be considered where relevant. Many cardiologists advise the use of coumarin rather than heparin as an anticoagulant for women with artificial valves. However, coumarin has a small risk of affecting the fetus which should be discussed fully.

Most women who have heart disease which is not causing them discomfort can be advised optimistically about having a properly supervised pregnancy and delivery. They should also be advised that in general there is little point putting off pregnancy, as it is unlikely that the heart disease will get any better. They should know that the pregnancy is going to be a greater hassle for them, for extra rest will be needed and physical activities will be curtailed. Similarly, after delivery, both in hospital and when they arrive home, extra rest may be required; one of the most important things will be to have a contingency plan to reorganize housework so that none or very little has to be done by the woman herself.

Raised Blood Pressure

A small number of women in the pregnancy age group have permanently raised blood pressure. Some have kidney disease; others have problems with the adrenal glands. Most, however, have no obvious underlying pathology and are labelled as having essential hypertension. Raised blood pressure affects the blood vessels in the brain, the action of the kidneys, and the efficiency of the heart; in consequence the aim of treating young people with hypertension is to keep the blood pressure within a reasonable range, if necessary by the use of drugs which lower high blood pressure.

A woman seeking prepregnancy care who has raised blood pressure has to be assessed thoroughly to check the degree of change in blood pressure and to see if it is in general within a range that is safe for herself and the baby. The heart and renal system must be checked and the use of anti-hypertensive drugs assessed. Generally speaking, if the woman's medical background is good, and the drugs are maintaining her blood pressure at a reasonable level, pregnancy will probably be safe for her and the child.

Case Study

Mrs K G was thirty-eight and she had two children already. She had been noted as having raised blood pressure and her General Practitioner was treating her for this with low doses of methyldopa. Having remarried two years before, her new husband was keen that they should have a child. However he was concerned about the effect it might have on her blood pressure and so Mr and Mrs G came to the prepregnancy clinic.

The report from the family doctor included the previous investigations done at another hospital when she started her treatment for raised blood pressure. We checked the function of the kidneys and the blood pressure. Since Mrs K G was well controlled, we advised her that it would probably be safe to proceed, under careful supervision.

Pregnancy followed six months later. Early on Mrs K G was very well but by twenty-two weeks, her blood pressure started to rise despite an increase in the methyldopa dosage. She was admitted to hospital where the treatment was changed to another anti-hypertensive agent, labetalol, which gave improved control of her blood pressure. After a few weeks Mrs K G was allowed out at weekends but even this was associated with a rise in blood pressure so she resigned herself to staying in hospital for the rest of her pregnancy.

We monitored the baby's growth and progress; with strict attention to blood pressure and the variation of drug dosage, Mrs K G got as far as thirty-four weeks of pregnancy. Then her blood pressure escaped our control despite even stronger measures and we had to deliver her by Caesarean section as an emergency. The baby girl weighed 1.8 kg (3 lb 14 oz) and required care at the neonatal unit for about four days. Despite the Caesarean section, Mrs K G was able to go to the neonatal unit each day to see her baby and on the fourth day they were both together back in the ward. Now Mrs K G has a thriving two-year-old child who is the darling of the family of three.

Most of the drugs used as anti-hypertensives have no effect on the fetus although they may be associated with changes in the blood flow to the uterus and therefore, in extreme cases, the supply of nutrients to the fetus later in pregnancy.

A serious complication may arise if pre-eclampsia is added to chronic raised blood pressure. Pre-eclampsia is a condition peculiar to pregnancy where there is an even greater rise in blood pressure accompanied by kidney damage, revealed when protein appears in the urine. This complication may go on to eclampsia, a condition where the mother experiences fits, or it can affect the unborn child by reducing the blood supply to the placental bed. This could lead to a reduction of nutrients in pregnancy and so produce a smaller baby; or it could reduce the supply of oxygen in labour. Clearly pre-eclampsia, when added to an already raised blood pressure, presents a serious problem for both the fetus and the mother.

The prepregnancy examination should check for organic changes in the heart or any evidence of deterioration of kidney function. If these are normal, then the blood pressure level should be assessed and the capacity of any anti-hypertensive drugs to maintain it at a reasonable level should be tested. If the woman is already on such therapeutic agents, the dosage may need to be adjusted.

The woman should be advised that in a subsequent pregnancy she will require much more rest during the daytime and may have to give up any work she is doing outside the home unless it is on a part-time basis and requires little physical exertion. She will require more frequent antenatal checks and special tests of fetal growth possibly involving visits to special hospital units which may be some distance from home. It is likely that she will need to be admitted to hospital in the last weeks of pregnancy. Couples need to remember that hypertension is not a temporary condition; childbearing should therefore be considered as soon as is reasonable and not put off until the woman is older, for by then the hypertension may be worse.

Kidney Disease

To maintain the balance of body functions, the kidneys have to excrete waste products at an efficient rate. Hence, the kidneys must be able to change their functional processes rapidly, sometimes to retain certain substances and at other times to excrete quickly. In chronic kidney disease, it is this inability to change excretory habits that is most serious.

During pregnancy there is strain on the kidneys. Blood flow is increased by up to 50% and so the clearance of waste products has to be even more efficient. An additional problem is that long-term kidney disease is often associated with raised blood pressure; in such cases all the problems described previously are added to the effects of the renal disease. If the blood pressure is normal, a woman with kidney problems has a much greater chance of achieving a successful outcome.

A woman with renal disease needs a full examination at the prepregnancy clinic, including a thorough assessment of the action of the kidneys. Further, any drug being taken for kidney disease must also be considered. Renal disease can change rapidly during pregnancy and so the woman must be prepared to rest more at home, or even to come into hospital. In an extreme case, pregnancy may have to be terminated in the first twenty weeks because of rapidly rising blood pressure or worsening renal function.

There are many different forms of renal disease, often related to chronic infection in youth, although some are associated with congenital abnormalities of the kidneys. The former are types of chronic pyelonephritis. If the infection is no longer active, a woman may pass through pregnancy with little change. Antibiotics may be required, but if renal function is fairly stable a reasonably good prognosis can be given. Those who have polycystic renal disease, a congenital disorder where a series of small cysts replace some of the excretory tissue of the kidney, usually know about it for it would have been diagnosed earlier. There is a risk of this condition being passed on to the child and so genetic counselling should be carried out before pregnancy. The parents should be warned that during pregnancy the fetal kidneys will have to be investigated using specific ultrasound in order to assess the possibility of inheritance in the unborn child.

An increasing number of women who have had a kidney transplant are now having families. The transplanted kidney is usually healthy but problems may arise because of the immunosuppressive drugs being given. These must be taken throughout the pregnancy, for otherwise the transplanted kidney may be rejected. The drugs may have some effect on the fetus, particularly in the early days, and the risks of this must be discussed.

The woman should also be warned that any serious deterioration of her renal function in the first six months of pregnancy may lead her doctor to advise termination. The transplanted kidney has often been sewn into the body low in the abdomen over the pelvic brim. This would interfere with a vaginal delivery and so a Caesarean section may be required.

Women in the pregnancy age group rarely have renal stones. For the few who do, if the renal stones are not causing symptoms before pregnancy, it is probable that pregnancy will proceed uneventfully. The most likely problem would be additional infection in the kidneys and this must be watched for carefully.

Acute Urinary Infections

Many women suffer from acute urinary infection during pregnancy because the bladder becomes more lax under the influence of the hormone progesterone. Bacteria ascend from the vagina up the urethra to colonize in the bladder or kidney, causing an infection. Usually the treatment is straightforward – antibiotics and an increased fluid intake. If a woman has had a urinary infection in a previous pregnancy, she would do well to consult the prepregnancy clinic before thinking about having another child.

A woman who has had several urinary infections in a previous pregnancy should be examined (before the next pregnancy) with X-rays and further bacteriological tests at the prepregnancy clinic in case there is a structural problem in the urinary tract. She should also be watched more carefully in another pregnancy; it would be wise to check a midstream specimen of urine early and to discuss plans in case of a sudden attack of urinary infection. These always seem to occur at five o'clock on a Sunday morning when one either cannot or does not wish to bother a doctor. Arrangements should therefore be made in the prepregnancy period. The woman should take extra fluids, which should be made slightly alkaline using sodium bicarbonate if necessary. It is also wise for her to keep a small quantity of one of the wide spectrum antibiotics at home so that she can start treatment straight away before medical help is available. These measures will greatly reduce the intensity and frequency of acute urinary infections in pregnancy.

Blood Diseases with Abnormal Haemoglobin

The blood circulating around the body carries oxygen to all tissues; the oxygen is transported by haemoglobin, a red pigment contained in red blood cells. This complex molecule has a strong affinity for oxygen, taking it up in the lungs, where there is a high concentration, and releasing it in the tissues, where the concentration of oxygen is low. If the structure of the haemoglobin molecule is changed, its binding capacity for oxygen will be impaired and the tissues will suffer from lack of oxygen.

The structure of the haemoglobin molecule is determined by chromosomes inherited from the father and mother and if this structure is altered, an inherited disease of haemoglobin abnormalities follows, a haemoglobinopathy. Many people with these abnormalities come from families originating in the Mediterranean basin, or from South-East Asia and Africa. The condition of haemoglobinopathy is recessive (see Chapter 4); this means that a woman can be a carrier for the condition without being affected herself. Many of us choose partners of a similar racial background, so a woman who is a carrier may well have children with a man who is himself well but has a recessive characteristic. By bringing together the two sets of recessive genes there is a 25% chance of producing a baby with a haemoglobin abnormality. Hence, there are two groups of people to be considered at the prepregnancy clinic: carriers and those with established conditions.

Structural Variations of Haemoglobin

The haemoglobin molecule consists of a massive number of amino acids; yet its function can be altered greatly by changing the order of even one of them, just as though a single brick had been mislaid and this changed the strength of a whole wall. In such haemoglobinopathies, the amino acid glutamine replaces a molecule of valine on one chain of the haemoglobin molecule. This small molecular substitution results in a distortion of the envelope of the red cell so that it looks like a crescent or sickle instead of the usual flattened dish shape.

If oxygen levels are reduced the red cells can sickle and stick in the small blood vessels, causing a narrowing or even a complete blockage. This leads to further oxygen deprivation so that the blood supply is cut off from the local areas. Such a sickling crisis is accompanied by severe pain which may occur in the limbs or in the abdomen. As well as low oxygen levels, dehydration and infection may lead to sickling crises and these too must be avoided. As mentioned in Chapter 4, sickling disorders are commonly found amongst Negro races.

Case Study

Miss V L and her partner, Mr J G, were both West Indians. She had been born in Kingston, Jamaica and came across to Britain at the age of two. Mr J G was from Trinidad and had come to Britain in his teens. They had met at a disco and some months later wanted to marry. However Miss V L's mother had told her that she had a blood disease and she 'could never carry children'. This naturally worried them both and since Miss V L's mother was now dead, there was no way of checking this matter further within the family. Miss V L's family doctor therefore advised her to come to the prepregnancy clinic.

Some simple tests were done on the blood of Miss V L and Mr J G. She was found to have a recessive sickle-cell trait, whilst his haemoglobin was perfectly normal in structure. They were advised that with a sickle-cell trait she would probably have a normal pregnancy and baby. She did not have sickle-cell disease but her child could carry the trait and thus be a carrier or even, unusually, actually have the disease.

Mr J G and Miss V L talked this over for a few weeks and decided to get married and go ahead with pregnancy. In fact the pregnancy went uneventfully and a girl weighing 3.4 kg (7 lb 9 oz) was born after thirty-nine weeks. On testing the baby's blood, she too was found to have sickle-cell trait but did not have the disease and Mrs V G was told of this so that she could warn her daughter in later life.

If the woman is a carrier of the condition (sickle-cell trait) she will probably have a normal pregnancy. Her haemoglobin should be checked before pregnancy; if a carrier state is found, her partner should also be checked. Should they both have the trait, the couple should be warned of the mathematical chances of having a child with sickle-cell disease. As well as the prepregnancy checking, further tests can be done on the fetus during early pregnancy by means of chorionic villus biopsy or, a little later, by taking a sample of fetal blood from the base of the umbilical cord to confirm whether or not the child is affected (see Chapter 4).

Sickle-cell disease in the mother can be a serious problem during pregnancy; there may be severe attacks in which the limbs swell with fluid as the red cells are broken down; blockage of blood vessels may lead to bouts of abdominal and joint pain which need careful surveillance. In addition, many of the problems of pregnancy, such as raised blood pressure, are increased and the fetus needs careful monitoring.

A woman who has sickle-cell disease should realize that it may be necessary to give up her usual work in the forthcoming pregnancy to rest at home; if that is not sufficient she will have to spend much time in hospital. She should always be close to medical care and be ready to report early small symptoms to her obstetricians and midwives. Blood transfusions may be required in extreme cases, and even exchange blood transfusions (where blood is exchanged with donor blood in a stepwise fashion to try to reduce the dangerous breakdown of red blood cells) are sometimes necessary in pregnancy. All this means being in the care of a maternity unit which includes an established blood transfusion (haematology) laboratory. Such expertise is found in only a few large hospitals, so the woman with sickle-cell disease may have to be admitted to hospital some distance from her home.

Any couple in which one partner has a family background of sickle-cell disease should seek prepregnancy counselling so that the haematological aspects may be worked out beforehand. There are now centres in Britain that specialize in sickle-cell disease, where doctors can give helpful advice and work out the correct odds. After such a consultation a couple may elect not to go for a pregnancy; or if they do, they will be aware of the problems that can arise and thus take measures in good time to ensure that the woman and her unborn child get the best care.

Haemoglobin Manufacture Faults

The haemoglobin molecule has two side-chains labelled alpha and beta; people from Mediterranean coastal regions may have a congenital change in the beta chain and so suffer from beta thalassaemia. If the molecular error is in the alpha side-chain it leads to alpha chain disease which is mainly found in people from South-East Asia. Like sickle-cell disease, thalassaemia can exist in the carrier state; the mother is not affected by the condition but if she marries someone with a similar chromosome defect, the child may be. Being a carrier is obviously not serious for the mother, but the disease state can be, particularly in pregnancy.

Beta thalassaemia can produce severe anaemia and congestive heart failure, and much extra care is required during pregnancy. Alpha thalassaemia, whilst it may produce some anaemia does not have such severe problems for the mother.

The carrier state again has less effect on the mother but ought to be diagnosed, particularly when considered in relation to the father's state.

The thalassaemias require careful prepregnancy assessment. Anaemia and crisis episodes are likely to be more frequent, and the fetus must be carefully monitored. Women should realize that they will probably have to give up paid work and have extra antenatal care. Admissions to hospital will also be more frequent, as they may require blood transfusion. Some obstetricians may even go so far as to advise against pregnancy for a woman with a beta thalassaemia, for the risks to the mother and to her unborn child are high. It must be stressed that the carrier states of either alpha or beta thalassaemia are not a particular risk to the mother or the baby in pregnancy. However, the mathematical chances of producing an affected child must be carefully worked out with geneticists in the prepregnancy period.

Hormonal Disorders

Diabetes

Since the introduction of insulin in the 1920s more diabetic women are leading normal lives, including becoming pregnant and producing healthy children. Before the advent of insulin young diabetics often did not even survive into the pregnancy age group; for those who did, the risks of childbirth to both mother and baby were so high that it was wise not to become pregnant. Since the 1950s the outlook has greatly improved. With good control, based on the frequent estimation of blood sugars, no diabetic mother need now fear that her condition will worsen (as it was once thought to) because of her pregnancy. The babies too are much better managed using a more rigid control of blood sugar. All this is based on prepregnancy care.

Case Study

Mrs A N was a twenty-nine-year-old diabetic who had been attending a diabetic clinic from the age of eleven. She was well stabilized on insulin and a moderately controlled diet. When she wanted to have a baby she came to the prepregnancy clinic beforehand where we outlined the potential problems and told her about possible treatments including hospital admission.

After a full assessment, including a series of blood sugar levels taken after meals, it became evident that she was not quite as stabilized as she thought; we checked her glycosylated haemoglobin which confirmed that her control should be stricter. The diabetic clinic and the diabetic dietitian worked hard with Mrs A N and achieved good control in about four months. Following that, she became pregnant.

There were problems in the first few weeks because, with her morning sickness, Mrs A N was unable to stick to her diet. In consequence she was giving herself more insulin than could be balanced by the carbohydrates she was taking in. She was admitted to hospital; her insulin-carbohydrate balance was restabilized and she was discharged at about fourteen weeks of pregnancy. After that Mrs A N did reasonably well but developed extra fluid in the uterus (polyhydramnios) and needed to be readmitted at thirty-four weeks' gestation. This settled down and we were about to discharge her when a blood pressure rise occurred. This continued despite bedrest; so, at thirty-seven weeks, labour was induced and after twelve hours of contractions Mrs A N produced a 4 kg (9 lb) infant who was healthy and well.

A large number of women have been found to have gestational diabetes, a potential diabetic phase which has no signs in ordinary life, but when stressed by pregnancy causes a woman to become a diabetic temporarily. Whilst the mother's outlook is good, the baby's is not, and such women should be detected and managed carefully through pregnancy, in order to have healthy children.

There are many problems which might arise in the unborn child if his diabetic mother is not cared for in an expert fashion. The first is the extra sugar which passes from the mother through the placenta and into the fetus during periods of instability. This stimulates the production of fetal insulin from the pancreas; fetal insulin is less efficient than the adult hormone and so the fetus lags behind the stimulation of extra sugar levels. This is associated with a faster growth rate; such increased growth can lead to babies which give trouble in labour and their size may make vaginal delivery impossible. The growth rate can be brought nearer to normal with rigid control of the mother's sugar/insulin balance, using frequent blood sugar estimations.

There is also an increase in the number of malformations in the offspring of diabetic mothers. The precise incidence varies with the control of diabetes at the time of conception, for it might be associated with fluctuations in blood sugar in very early pregnancy. In general, fetal abnormalities tend to be more severe and several may be found in one baby. However, this risk can be reduced by preparation in the prepregnancy period.

A diabetic woman should take careful prepregnancy advice to ensure her fitness for pregnancy. In particular, the more serious side effects of diabetes must be excluded before pregnancy is contemplated; potential damage to the heart, kidneys and retina of the eye should be assessed for it is these organs that could be affected if the diabetes worsens. Those with such damage already may be advised against pregnancy. Women who are not so affected should be assessed to ensure that these serious complications are not likely to be speeded up by pregnancy.

It is important that women and their partners are instructed at the prepregnancy clinic about the frequent self-testing of blood sugar which is required in pregnancy. Urine testing is not precise enough to follow a pregnant diabetic. The changed monitoring process during pregnancy will involve much effort and concentration on the part of the mother to read her blood sugar tests herself and to adjust her insulin dosage. This needs time to sort out and early pregnancy is too short a time zone; it must be a prepregnancy task.

The combination of glucose with one of the limbs of the haemoglobin molecule (glycosylated haemoglobin) can be measured in the blood; it reflects the variation of blood glucose levels in the previous six weeks. Thus, the measurement of glycosylated haemoglobin provides a guide to the woman's control of her sugar/insulin balance. It should be checked in the prepregnancy clinic and used as a guide for any restabilization of insulin that may be required. This is probably the most important single biochemical test that can be done in the prepregnancy clinic for the diabetic mother-to-be.

It is important to plan a pregnancy at a time when the diabetic mother can give maximum attention to any prepregnancy clinical advice she has been given. Contraception should be used until that time is reached and then the pregnancy can be started. There might be discussion in the prepregnancy clinic about later sterilization. Such discussion should be carefully related to the individual woman's age, the medical complications of the diabetes, the size of her family, and the wishes of both partners.

By seeing a woman at a prepregnancy clinic, it is possible to improve diabetic control in the first weeks of pregnancy. This is important for it is at this time that abnormalities are laid down. A research worker in East Germany examined 292 diabetics who he had only seen after the eighth week of pregnancy, and found a 7.5% malformation rate; whereas 128 diabetic women who attended his prepregnancy clinic and were seen early had only 0.8% malformations. These sorts of figures indicate the importance of prepregnancy consultation for a diabetic.

It is important that the diabetic woman be warned of the need to be precise in the timing of her pregnancy. She should keep a calendar of her menstrual dates, and a pregnancy test should be performed as soon as suspicion exists. Whilst ultrasound can be used later on, it is sometimes less precise in measuring the fetus of a diabetic mother than that of another woman. An additional benefit of prepregnancy consultation with the diabetic mother is that she can have all the checks for German measles and haemoglobinopathies performed early to exclude other possible causes of problems. Advice about diet should also be given at this time.

Many couples attending for prepregnancy care want to know about the chances of diabetes being passed on to their future child. The risk is very small; if the woman's partner is not diabetic the odds are about 1%. However, diabetics tend to meet each other in youth and a higher proportion than background marry each other; they understand each other's problems and are sympathetic towards each other's way of life. In such circumstances, where both parents are diabetic, the risk of having diabetic offspring rises to about 5%.

Thyroid Disorders

Overactivity of the thyroid gland is quite common in the pregnancy age group, with up to 5% of women being affected. Unless they receive effective treatment for the hyperactivity, these women will be infertile. However, with proper and effective treatment of the thyroid problem, their conception rates are as good as those of other women. During pregnancy it is quite unusual to be able to diagnose a new case of overactive thyroid disease, for all the results of the investigations are changed by the pregnancy itself.

Underactive thyroid disease is less usual in women of the pregnancy age group. When it occurs and is not treated, there is usually a lack of ovulation, making pregnancy impossible. If the condition is corrected with replacement thyroid hormones, then the woman is normally in a good state to go through pregnancy. The exact dosage of thyroid hormone may need to be altered during pregnancy, but it is unlikely to have any harmful effect on the unborn child, and most do very well.

Anti-thyroid drugs can themselves be responsible for problems in pregnancy. Carbimazole has now been used for long enough that it can be safely said not to carry any increased risk of producing fetal abnormalities. It may, however, cause some depression in the fetal thyroid gland; the baby should therefore be examined carefully after the delivery in case he or she requires extra thyroid hormone. If a woman has been treated with radioactive iodine, it would theoretically be possible for the radioactivity to affect the fetal thyroid gland. In such a case it would be wise to wait for about a year after the last radioactive therapy has been given before trying for pregnancy.

During pregnancy the dosage of the woman's anti-thyroid drugs may need to be altered; this is not predictable and so she should receive extra and more frequent antenatal care. Blood levels of the thyroid-stimulating hormones should be checked at the prepregnancy clinic, for some women with overactive thyroid glands may have antibodies which could cross the placenta. If such antibodies are found, the woman should be told that the fetus might be affected, and a careful check should be made immediately after delivery. Whilst the baby is in the uterus he is usually in good health.

Adrenal Gland Disorders

Previously women who had suppression of the adrenal glands used not to become pregnant but now, with replacement therapy from corticosteroids, they are becoming so at a normal rate. They usually have a normal pregnancy but will need extra antenatal care; the growth of the baby should be checked during pregnancy with ultrasound. Extra cortisone* will be required in labour.

Women with increased adrenal activity (adrenal hyperplasia) have usually been diagnosed before pregnancy and the maintenance dose of hormones has been decided. Such women do not tend to ovulate unless this hormonal correction puts them into a normal hormone balance. After treatment most of them have a normal pregnancy, although the risk of raised blood pressure is slightly higher than usual, even with well-balanced treatment.

Respiratory Disorders

Asthma

Amongst women in the pregnancy age group, the most common respiratory problem is asthma. For a variety of reasons, the small airways in the lungs go into spasm, making it difficult for the woman to breathe out. This is distressing and may lead to retention of lung secretions so that chest infections can follow asthmatic attacks. The usual treatment is inhalation of bronchial dilator drugs to relax the airtubes, and steroids* taken by mouth.

There seems to be little excess risk to the fetus from a mother with asthma, even if she is receiving steroids. However, the baby may be slightly smaller than usual. The mother will probably require extra steroids at the time of delivery since her own manufacture of this hormone might be depressed by the extra steroids she is being given. Injections of bronchial dilators, such as theophylline, can be used in pregnancy without any adverse effects on the embryo.

Case Study

Miss R P was a medical social worker. She was a tense, hardworking woman who had suffered from asthma since childhood. Most of these attacks were controlled with an inhaler but occasionally, when under stress at work, she needed injections to overcome the spasm in her chest.

She came to the prepregnancy clinic to discuss in general what might happen if she became pregnant. She

(Case Study cont.)

was frightened that the baby growing in the uterus would push up on the diaphragm and she would not be able to breathe. She was not actually contemplating marriage or childbirth at the time but wanted to know in general what the outlook was.

A simple physical examination and chest X-ray showed no obvious structural impairment of the lungs. We then discussed the events of pregnancy from conception to a few weeks after childbirth, pointing out the aspects of asthma and its treatment which might affect pregnancy, as well as where pregnancy might affect the asthma. This was a long interview but Miss R P was very receptive and made notes throughout, jotting down the various points.

We did not see Miss R P again but she wrote to us three years later saying that she was now settled in Wales and had a child. She had found the interview in the prepregnancy clinic most reassuring; none of the worst things discussed had happened but at least she knew what might occur and what management might be available. It is even possible that the prepregnancy interview may itself have helped to prevent some of the more serious aspects of the asthma by lessening her anxiety.

The effect of pregnancy on asthma is very varied. In one big study at Queen Charlotte's Hospital, London, half the pregnant women showed no change, a quarter improved, and the other quarter got worse. There is therefore no reason to advise a woman with asthma not to get pregnant. Some get asthma in response to external irritants such as pollens; if delivery could be planned away from the pollen season, this would obviously be sensible.

The harmful effects of smoking cigarettes on top of asthma should not need emphasizing but the prepregnancy clinic may be another place where the woman can be warned of this.

At a prepregnancy clinic a woman with asthma should

be assessed for the degree of asthma she suffers, and asked for her details of medication. She can be reassured that some women with asthma actually improve because their bodies manufacture more cortisone; their babies are usually normal.

Tuberculosis

Tuberculosis is now unusual in most of the population in the pregnancy age group in the United Kingdom, although in certain groups, like the Gujarati Indians and some of the West Indians, the incidence is higher than for a UK background.

Normally tuberculosis does not affect the pregnancy, nor does the pregnancy particularly accelerate progress of the disease. These days women with tuberculosis in the United Kingdom become pregnant whilst on treatment, and this medication should be carefully assessed in the prepregnancy clinic. Some of the drugs used (such as ethambutol and isoniazid) are perfectly safe for the fetus. Streptomycin, however, might cause damage to the hearing of the unborn child, and rifampicin has been reported to be associated with severe congenital defects, as has ethionamide. A new anti-tuberculous drug, pyrazinamide, is not associated with such abnormalities.

Most women know which drugs they are on, and so the prepregnancy counsellor can discuss with the consultant in charge of their tuberculosis management which medicines would be best when starting the pregnancy and in the first few months of pregnancy. After the fetus is formed, in the first fourteen weeks, the fuller spectrum of antibiotics can be used, but in the early months it would be wise to avoid those drugs known to be associated with fetal problems.

If a woman with treated pulmonary tuberculosis becomes pregnant and stays under the controlled care of a tuberculosis physician and an obstetrician, there is no evidence that her condition will deteriorate. The baby may have to be isolated from the mother if there are still active tubercle bacilli in her sputum but this is very rare. The infant can be inoculated against tuberculosis as early as six weeks old.

Cystic Fibrosis

This respiratory condition is not commonly found in young mothers, but as treatment in childhood improves, more women with this condition are appearing in the pregnancy age group. The principal reason for obtaining prepregnancy advice is that many women are very frightened of producing a baby who has cystic fibrosis.

Case Study

Mrs J F had had two children before; they were now aged six and two. The first was normal but the second had moderately severe cystic fibrosis which affected the child's lungs. Mrs J F was worried about the possibility of this occurring in another baby. We told her what could be done with an amniocentesis* test and we discussed this in great detail.

When, eight months later, she came to see us in early pregnancy, she naturally asked for these tests and we did them. We were pleased to assure her that there was no evidence of cystic fibrosis enzymes in the current pregnancy. This naturally gave her a much happier time during pregnancy and labour. When we tested her child a few days after birth we found her to be unaffected. That child is now four years old and has subsequently developed normally with no problems.

Inheritance is by a recessive pattern. If a woman with the condition marries a man without it, there is a 1 in 4 chance of producing a baby with cystic fibrosis. Hence, it depends on the degree to which the mother's chromosomes and those of her partner are affected. If all the chromosomes in the egg or sperm carry the trait, that person is homozygous (they pass the characteristics on every time they reproduce). In some people only half the gametes bear the affected chromosome. Such people are described as heterozygous. The risks of passing on the condition are shown opposite.

Risks of Incidence of Cystic Fibrosis

		Woman	
	Normal	Heterozygous CF	Homozygous CF
Normal	0	0	0
Partner Heterozygous	0	25%	50%
Homozygous	0	50%	100%

(0 = very small background risk – less than 1%)

It might be thought that the chances were slim of those with such an unusual condition meeting and having children. However, those with a chronic physical condition often choose a partner with a similar problem for they are able to give each other support and sympathy. Such women therefore appear disproportionately often in the prepregnancy clinic with an affected partner.

A woman with cystic fibrosis should be checked very carefully before pregnancy. Some sufferers may have such severe respiratory problems that it would be unwise for them to become pregnant; if this is the case it must be stated. Amongst other women, the condition of the lungs may have affected the heart, causing early decompensation of the circulation leading to mild heart failure and poor oxygenation of the blood passing to the body. Yet another group may get uncontrollable recurrent chest infections, the frequency and intensity of which could increase in pregnancy. It would be wise for a respiratory physician, in conjunction with the prepregnancy clinic, to make a special assessment, including the levels of oxygen transported in the blood and a full check of the respiratory tract.

The woman and her partner may be told of tests that can be performed in early pregnancy to check whether the embryo is affected with cystic fibrosis. These can be either an amniocentesis done at sixteen weeks, when a chemical test is performed on the enzymes present in the fetal cells, or, at specialist hospitals, a direct assessment of fetal cells taken by chorionic villus* sampling performed at ten weeks. These tests are improving each year and by the early 1990s should be safe and reasonably predictable.

Anyone with cystic fibrosis will have been advised of the adverse effect of cigarette smoking. The prepregnancy clinic may be the place to reinforce this warning for the woman is now beginning to think of two people – herself and her unborn child.

When all these aspects have been discussed, the woman and her partner can make a more informed decision, rather than automatically assuming that all those who have had a baby with cystic fibrosis should avoid pregnancy in the future.

Sarcoidosis of the Lung

This condition is unusual in the pregnancy age group, but women do appear in the prepregnancy clinic more often than background because of referrals from respiratory specialists. Generally sarcoidosis improves during pregnancy, probably because of the increase in circulating corticosteroids from the mother's adrenal glands; the situation may however deteriorate afterwards.

The degree to which sarcoidosis affects the respiratory tract should be assessed carefully by the respiratory physician and the prepregnancy obstetrician. After clinical examination, X-rays and respiratory function tests, an opinion should be offered to the woman. Generally the advice is to go ahead, as the pregnancy and the unborn child are unlikely to be affected.

Epilepsy

This is the most common neurological condition found in the pregnancy age group, affecting about 1 in 200 women. Most have already been diagnosed and put on anti-convulsant treatment. Pregnancy may make the condition of epilepsy worse overall. While half the women will be unaffected and 10% will have fewer seizures, 40% will have an increased rate of fitting, especially if they are not taking anti-epileptic drugs.

In the prepregnancy period the frequency and severity of fits should be carefully assessed. This information should be related to the already existing drug therapy and details of the medication should be determined accurately. It is possible to measure the level of the drugs in the blood during pregnancy and this may be considered valuable when advising about future treatment, especially in the early weeks of pregnancy.

All anti-convulsant drugs have an effect on the unborn child and have been linked with extra risks of malformations. Irrespective of any drugs, parents with epilepsy have a higher risk of producing babies with malformation, and so there is a double set of variables. Epileptic women with virtually no seizures, who do not require anti-epileptic drugs, have a risk factor ×2 of having a baby with a malformation over the risk to a non-epileptic woman. If drugs are needed to control the epilepsy there is an even higher risk; in the greatest risk category for malformed babies are those women who still have seizures despite taking medication. In their case the risk factor is ×12.

Hence, if a woman with epilepsy wants advice about a future pregnancy, once the frequency and severity of fits have been assessed, the possibility of stopping drugs before and in very early pregnancy should be considered carefully. The frequency of fitting in early pregnancy will relate to the pattern of fits in the last year. The effect of pregnancy on fit frequency varies enormously in different women, ranging from a significant increase to a great reduction; the prepregnancy pattern of fits returns when the baby is born. If a neurologist at the prepregnancy consultation considers that the woman's fits are so frequent that she needs to continue anti-epileptic medication, she should be warned of the possibility of the baby being affected.

The most common congenital abnormality associated with

all anti-epileptic drugs is hare lip or cleft palate. Sodium valproate is especially associated with neural tube defects, and trimethadione is linked with cleft palate, low-set ears, irregular teeth and speech disturbance. Both these drugs should be avoided if possible by women contemplating pregnancy and other anti-epileptic drugs should be used for those who need them.

At the prepregnancy clinic the woman's background neurological state, the drugs she is taking and their beneficial effect must be balanced against her fear of continuing to take drugs she believes to be potentially harmful to the fetus. This difficult issue requires careful individual attention. Further, the mother-to-be should be warned that many anti-epileptic drugs prevent the absorption of the vitamin folic acid and so extra folate tablets should be given during pregnancy to help the fetus to grow properly.

It may take some months to wean the woman from her long-standing anti-epileptic drug, and she must be made well aware of the potential risks of recurrent seizures during this time. For instance, she should be warned of the dangers of falling in inappropriate places such as fires. In addition the Vehicle Licensing Centre in Swansea should be notified that she is changing her status as an epileptic, for the anti-epileptic drug withdrawal may affect her ability to drive.

Epilepsy is one of the areas where prepregnancy consultation can be very beneficial; the background condition itself can be distinguished from the therapies given long before pregnancy starts. The counsellor can then warn the couple of the possibility of the various combinations of problems.

Alimentary Tract Disorders

Peptic Ulceration
This often occurs among women of the pregnancy age group. In general, peptic ulcers tend to improve a little in pregnancy,

due partly to a reduction of the acid secretion, and partly to the protective effects of the hormone oestrogen. However, mild irritation of either the oesophagus (the gullet) or the duodenum (the upper part of the intestine) may occur, due to reflux or overflow respectively, causing the acid gastric secretions to appear in the wrong place. These are not serious conditions and pregnancy can proceed with the help of gentle antacids.

Crohn's Disease and Ulcerative Colitis

These inflammatory conditions of the lower small intestine and the large intestine are often associated with a reduced fertility, but with the treatments being offered these days fertility returns to normal. These drugs do not usually affect the unborn child even if the mother is taking them when the pregnancy starts. Prepregnancy counselling should include careful assessment of the present state of the bowel and the medication the woman is receiving; this is usually Salazopyrine and one of the corticosteroids. Both these groups of drugs are relatively safe in pregnancy.

The effect of the pregnancy on the bowel disease will, however, need careful monitoring; there may be remissions of the inflammation in the bowel but this does not seem to occur any more often than in women who are not pregnant. There should be close cooperation with a gastroenterologist at the prepregnancy clinic, and the woman can usually be given an optimistic prognosis.

A few women have previously had bowel resections (removal of the bowel), and these operations may have led to adhesions in the abdominal cavity. The adhesions could affect the Fallopian tubes by kinking them, making it more difficult to become pregnant; once that has been achieved, adhesions do not usually affect the progress of pregnancy seriously but they can be a nuisance. As the uterus with its growing contents rises up out of the pelvis, it may stretch some of the adhesions, causing transient pain. If the woman requires a Caesarean section, this can be done readily, for the adhesions are usually pushed out of the way by the growing uterus. The major problem in the operation is that any adhesions between the bladder and the uterus can give the surgeon great difficulty. For this reason, a more experienced obstetrician should be chosen for a Caesarean section in these circumstances. However, the general advice still stands that whilst they are uncomfortable, the presence of adhesions *per se* should not be a reason for a woman not to go for pregnancy.

Liver Diseases

These are fairly common in the pregnancy age group. This is a complex field and an expert hepatologist needs to be consulted at the prepregnancy stage. Some liver conditions (acute fatty liver in pregnancy) are likely to flare up, making the woman very ill and affecting the baby. Hence, if there is a history of a serious attack of this in a previous pregnancy it may be wise not to have another baby. In other conditions, the outcome for mother and child will depend more on the degree of liver damage than the precise disease itself.

Careful prepregnancy tests must be done on the liver assessing its function. If there is only slight impairment of liver function the pregnancy will probably be normal. The more severe the damage, the more likely there are to be problems both for the fetus and the mother; in certain situations it may be necessary to advise the mother to avoid pregnancy. In borderline cases the woman should be warned that, should a pregnancy start and the function of the liver deteriorate, an abortion may have to be carried out in the first half of pregnancy to save the mother's health.

AIDS

This is a relatively new viral disease which has had a huge impact on the public's imagination. It is spread by direct contact from the blood of an infected person to the blood of the recipient. It can be passed on through blood transfusions or blood products from donors if these have not been screened; in the United Kingdom this is always done most meticulously. It can also be spread by infected and non-infected people sharing intravenous needles used in drug-taking. Less commonly for women, AIDS can be passed on by violent sexual intercourse, particularly if a break is made in the skin; thus anal intercourse is the most likely way of spreading this disease sexually rather than vaginal intercourse.

In Britain far fewer women are affected than men. In February 1990 there were over 2,898 men with AIDS as opposed to 123 women. In consequence, it is not a common condition in pregnancy but is greatly feared because of the lack of any effective cure.

Any woman who thinks she has AIDS would do well to have this checked by a simple blood test before she considers pregnancy. There may be a risk if her partner is bisexual, if she has shared intravenous needles in drug-taking, or if she has had a blood transfusion in a foreign country. Some women who come from the middle belt of Africa may have contracted AIDS from their partners, for it is far more common in that part of the world. Women in these groups should consult the prepregnancy clinic for advice. A blood test can be performed and this gives some reassurance if antibodies are not found. However, it takes two or three months for antibodies to develop fully and so the tests may have to be repeated.

If a woman who is infected becomes pregnant, there is a risk of affecting the unborn child through the placenta. The exact risk is not known but probably between one-fifth and one-third of babies born to mothers with AIDS show AIDS antibodies in their blood. In some cases this may indicate a spill-over of antibodies from the mother and not a real infection of the baby, but still the risk is there. We are less certain about the risks of infection from a mother's milk after delivery; risks of this must be considered individually. At present there is no vaccine or drug to treat AIDS but work is proceeding rapidly in many parts of the world and there may be one in a few years' time.

Psychiatric Disorders

We all live in a spectrum of behaviour which usually ranges around completely normal; at each end of that spectrum are full blown psychiatric disorders such as depression or mania. Generally we stay in the normal range, but we can easily slip from this middle ground into behaving irrationally. If this is only a temporary aberration of violent temper or mild depression it is not usually considered to be a psychiatric problem; it passes as the environment changes. However, if it continues, with delusions on the one hand or deep gloom on the other, psychiatric help is required.

In pregnancy many such conditions are made worse by the hormonal changes in the woman's body. It is wise for any woman with a pre-existing psychological problem to consult her prepregnancy clinic in order to go through the details of what may happen in a subsequent pregnancy. Further, the care of the baby after delivery has to be considered if the woman is likely to go through long-term psychological illness.

Many of the drugs given in psychological treatment cross the placenta and could affect the baby. There are so many of these that it would be hard to particularize them in a chapter like this. A woman who is on medication for psychiatric disorder should consult her advisers, in conjunction with the prepregnancy clinic, as to how the pregnancy may affect the disease, and conversely how the disease and the drugs being given to treat it may affect the pregnancy.

Conclusions

All these illnesses may sound very severe but in fact they affect only a small proportion of women who wish to get pregnant. It is important, however, for those in this group to get specific advice, and here the specialist prepregnancy clinic is useful. The prepregnancy counsellor may not know about every aspect of medicine but he or she will have built up contacts with physicians and surgeons interested in particular aspects of these diseases in pregnancy. The counsellor can then contact these specialists and refer the woman to them for advice.

It is essential that any woman with a pre-existing medical condition thinks very carefully about pregnancy and consults with a prepregnancy doctor and the specialist concerned, for knowledge in all these fields is advancing rapidly. One should never rely on the information of five years ago nor that of well-meaning friends or relatives. On the whole, more and more women with serious illnesses are going through pregnancy with good results. Ten years ago women who had artificial heart valves would not have considered becoming pregnant, but now so many have done so that there is a substantial and growing body of knowledge on the subject. At prepregnancy clinics women can be given advice about all sorts of conditions – advice based on good experience. In the end it is always better to consult and ask, rather than bury one's head in the sand.

SEVEN

Work

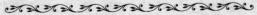

That ever God ordained men and women to live idly, I never yet read or heard; and Lycurgus, that famous Spartan commander, being asked the reason why he forced young virgins to labour, answered very wisely and discreetly, that thereby cleansing their bodies of evil excrements, they might bring forward lusty children when they were married.

Culpeper

Many more women are now working during pregnancy; they are also continuing to work until much closer to the time of expected birth. Just after the Second World War, about half of all working women continued their jobs into pregnancy and the vast majority of them gave up by about the twenty-eighth week. In a more recent study, three-quarters of working women were continuing into pregnancy and most of them going on to thirty-six or even thirty-eight weeks. This great change in women's attitudes towards working in pregnancy, and its reluctant acceptance by employers and legislators, is one of the revolutions of the 1970s and 1980s.

These days most couples plan on two incomes coming into the household. The size of a mortgage is usually based upon the total income of both partners and repayments demand that two wage packets continue to come in. In the first few years before a family starts expenditure on household goods and leisure activities is also based on double income: cars, furniture and overseas holidays, to name but a few examples. When a woman becomes pregnant, although a maternity grant is paid (see Box opposite), she is suddenly faced with the prospect of having to give up work for some time; many women now are reluctant to start that break too early. They would like to go on working into pregnancy; they feel that pregnancy is a normal event and they wish to earn income while they can. Further, they wish to have more of their statutory maternity leave after childbirth so that they can spend more time getting to know their newborn baby.

Pregnancy Entitlements

Pregnant women resident in the United Kingdom are entitled to a series of benefits. These change from time to time so precise details cannot be given here. Up-to-date information can always be obtained from your local Social Security office or from the Medical Social Workers' Department of the hospital you are attending for antenatal care.

Maternity Grant

This is a single payment paid by cheque. It can generally be claimed after the twenty-sixth week of pregnancy by a woman who has lived in the United Kingdom for six of the last twelve months before her baby is due.

Maternity Allowance

This is a weekly payment through the Post Office for eighteen weeks, usually starting at about twenty-nine weeks of pregnancy. Qualification depends upon your previous National Insurance contributions or credits. Claim forms are available from the Social Security Office or the Antenatal Clinic.

Maternity Pay

This comes from your employer and not Social Security. It should be equivalent to 90% of your basic pay for the first six weeks of your maternity leave.

Maternity Leave

Leave can be taken from the twenty-ninth week of pregnancy and can go on up to twenty-nine weeks after the birth of the baby, even though that birth may not be exactly on time. Usually you have the right to return to your old job, provided you have informed your employer of your intention to come back. Certain firms are too small to apply this rule and in some cases you may not have worked there long enough. Details are available from your Union representative or your company's Personnel Department.

(Pregnancy Entitlements cont.)

Other Maternity Rights

All pregnant women are entitled to free milk and vitamins, free prescriptions and free dental treatment for up
to one year after the child is born. A woman is entitled
to take time off work to attend antenatal care, provided
she informs her employer of the appointment. In certain
circumstances, if the total family income is low, travelling
expenses can be claimed for these visits.

The other reason for working on into pregnancy is that the
years of reproduction in this country are exactly the same as
those in which we all advance in our business or profession.
What we have achieved by the age of thirty-five is usually an
indication of our life's career potential, and yet it is also the
years from twenty to thirty-five in which women tend to have
children. In this context, every pregnancy is seen as a minor
gap in advancement and so these gaps are reduced as far as
possible in order to continue an occupation for profit, interest
or ambition.

If you leave your job in pregnancy, you are usually entitled
to have your job back with the same employer after maternity
leave. This applies if he or she employs more than five people
and you have been working for two years in your usual job
or longer in a part-time job. If you wish to protect your job
you must give your employer twenty-one days notice of your
intention to stop working and you cannot leave your job before
the twenty-ninth week of pregnancy. In return, your employer
must keep your job open for a year and offer it to you when
you say you wish to return. That exact job may have gone but
'a job of equivalent nature' must be provided. In these days
of industrial uncertainty it is often a comfort to women who
are giving up their work for pregnancy to feel that their
decision will not imperil their capacity to work in the future if
they want to.

Types of Work

For those women who run households, housework must always be considered first when examining problems before and in early pregnancy. In the house there are the duties of cleaning, cooking, washing and the loads imposed by other children, by husbands and maybe by parents. There are no days off for sick leave, there is no rest room and no relief by coming in late to work. It is the constant load that many women accept when they marry, and it is often assumed by the male that housework will continue even though paid work outside the home may be added to the load.

In the home there are the problems of fatigue, which we will consider later, and a few specific problems involving the chemicals used in washing and painting. Tiredness is the major problem in housework; that and boredom can significantly influence the outcome of pregnancy if they act in extreme.

Case Study

Mrs T.A had previously lost four pregnancies between sixteen and twenty-four weeks and came to the prepregnancy clinic for advice about a possible future pregnancy.

Amongst our enquiries we asked about her work. She said she did none but we enquired a little further and asked if she worked at home. She replied: 'Oh yes, but that does not count.' Further enquiry showed that as well as coping with a husband she kept house for an aged mother and father and for an elder brother who was affected by Down's Syndrome. She would get up at 6 a.m. to do all the housework in a rather large, inefficient Victorian house in South London. This would include taking breakfast in bed to two members of the family. She would then shop for the five adults who lived in the house, do all the cleaning herself with no help, prepare lunch and

(Case Study cont.)

an evening meal for five. She took it upon herself to do all the decorating in this Victorian mausoleum and rarely stopped work until 10 p.m. She might watch the news on television before dropping exhausted into bed, to start the next day at 6 a.m.

When we pointed out that this was work, and far harder than most people do in their paid workplace, Mrs T A took a while to absorb what we were saying; she felt it was her responsibility in life to do this. Slowly, however, we persuaded her. When she came to see us before her next pregnancy she was receptive to our advice to rest in early pregnancy; the easiest way was not to do all the household tasks she did. It caused a minor revolution at home but eventually others did join in and her workload was lessened. Mrs T A happily delivered a 2.8 kg (6 lb 3 oz) boy at thirty-eight weeks of gestation.

Outside the home, there is a great variety of work a woman can do but in actuality most are in a narrow range of working practices. Of the ten million women working in the United Kingdom in 1985, three million worked in offices, two million in service jobs and one million in health or education. Some of these are physically easy jobs but others involve strenuous activities, although few women go so far as those in the Soviet Union or the USA by becoming coalminers or steelworkers. Women also tend to do a greater proportion of part-time work than men; although the activity may be great, they might therefore spend fewer hours doing it.

However many hours are spent at work, an important factor is travelling to and from your workplace. If you live in a small village and can cycle five minutes to your work and five minutes home in the evening, that is a pleasure (except on wet days). Unfortunately most women live in large conurbations and travel for an hour or so in the morning and the evening in crowded rush hour trains, buses and tubes. The noise, stress, and in some cases smoke from other people's tobacco can be most unpleasant. It was a great health advance when the London Underground system abolished cigarette smoking in all stations and trains. The numbers of non-smoking carriages are increasing greatly on British Rail and segregation on buses is becoming more favourable to the non-smoker.

Despite these moves, travel is still stressful. Studies performed in Spain have shown that the likelihood of preterm labour increases greatly with the amount of stressful public travel a woman has to suffer in her daily round. Try to work to flexitime if your job is in a big city with rush hours. Your employer may be happy to let you change your hours slightly to avoid rush hour travel if he or she is approached before a pregnancy. This would allow a slightly less stressful journey to work and so less fatigue.

Case Study

Mrs M S was a barrister who had suffered from asthma since childhood. It was now in a moderate phase, being controlled by inhalations and occasional treatment with steroids. She had been pregnant previously but had miscarried at fourteen weeks. She attributed this to a recurrence of her asthma when she became very breathless, leading to a prolonged, productive cough. She wanted therefore to avoid anything that might cause the asthma to recur.

At the prepregnancy clinic we made some enquiries and found that she was not particularly susceptible to any of the pollens so the asthma was not seasonal. Asking about her work, she told us that she lived in Reigate and worked in the City of London; her journey to work each day was about fifty-five minutes on an extremely smoky train. When we pointed out the unpleasantness of this, almost two hours of exposure to other people's exhaled smoke, she remembered how much better she had felt

(Case Study cont.)

when she was on holiday in her parents' home in Wales and not exposed to this secondary smoking.

Mrs M S considered our advice so important that she reorganized her life and took a partnership with a firm of solicitors in Reigate. She then found she could walk to work (two and a half minutes) and could do her shopping in the lunch hour. This shortened her day considerably and she was delighted. Further, when she did get pregnant she had no recurrence of asthma and happily delivered a 3.7 kg (8 lb 4 oz) boy at thirty-nine weeks.

Hazards at Work

There is a wide variety of hazards at work which may impinge on a woman who is pregnant; these should be known about before pregnancy starts so that she can make an informed choice about her own work. They may be divided into specific hazards, usually physically toxic, and the non-specific ones of fatigue and tiredness.

Specific Hazards

These toxic hazards are mostly those that cause alterations in the cells of the growing embryo so that congenital abnormalities are produced. As discussed in Chapter 2, during the first ten weeks of the embryo's life any chemical, physical or infectious hazard can cause a specific change, depending upon the stage of development. In addition, exposure to the same or similar stimulus later on can sometimes slow down the rate of intrauterine growth, producing a small-for-dates baby. Specific hazards may be divided into physical, chemical and biological hazards.

PHYSICAL HAZARDS

X-rays are a risk to women in early pregnancy. This is well known to those who work in radiological departments in hospitals or deal with radioisotopes in laboratories. However, fewer people realize that X-ray machines can be used in the examination of postal packages in many large firms or until recently to examine children's feet in shoe shops. Whilst these have mostly been regulated in Britain, in many parts of the world X-rays are still used relatively indiscriminately. The dose may be very low for the individual person buying shoes but it could accumulate and present a much higher risk for someone working in that shop.

Ultrasound is widely used in laboratories and industry as well as in diagnostic obstetrics. In the last decade fears about ultrasound have been mostly assuaged. Firstly the energy output of the amount of ultrasound involved is minute. Further, there is no epidemiological evidence that ultrasound is associated with any abnormalities or defects of the human species. Probably some fifty million women have used ultrasound in early pregnancy and as yet no pattern of resultant problems in the newborn has shown itself. Strictly speaking, one cannot yet be absolutely certain for we have only been using ultrasound for twenty years, but so far no hazard has turned up. Women need not be too upset if they work with ultrasound or have ultrasound tests on their unborn child. Considering the benefits of ultrasound, it is unlikely that any resultant hazard to the fetus would now be discovered which would outweigh the advantages of this method in obstetrics.

Another scare was raised when many secretaries began to use visual display units (VDUs). Several reports appeared in the late 1970s about small groups of women working with VDUs who showed a high rate of pregnancy loss. Of ten women who became pregnant in a given site using VDUs, a majority might have either miscarried or had preterm labours. This led to a great fear of the VDU which is probably mostly unnecessary. An example was the Sears Roebuck Cluster in Dallas; there 75 women in one department were using VDUs and 12 became pregnant. Seven of those pregnancies ended in miscarriage and there was one neonatal death. Hence, the failure rate in this group would be 8 in 12 (67%); by contrast, in a group of 49 workers in the same firm working in departments not using VDUs, there was a 15% failure rate. These differences may seem highly significant but because the numbers are small they cannot be taken as applying to other places, nor indeed can one particularly blame the VDUs.

There were over ten million VDUs in use in the USA and a million and a half in the United Kingdom in 1987. If we estimate the number of groups of more than ten women who are using these, there will be 20,000 groups. If we allow a mean figure for a natural pregnancy failure rate of 15%, then by the distribution of numbers by chance, in 29 of these 20,000 units, there will be clusters containing more than half the pregnant women experiencing a pregnancy failure each year. This is the natural mathematics of distribution curves and nothing to do with the VDU. Of course there will also be another 29 clusters among the total number of groups who have a 0% failure rate but they will probably not be reported.

A large questionnaire study, done in Canada in 1986, looked at 52,000 hospitalized deliveries and showed that the malformation rate in the VDU group was 3.3% compared with 3.7% in the non-user group. Neither the abnormality rate nor that of miscarriages varied significantly with the different levels of use. Other studies from Finland, Sweden and the USA confirm this so probably fears are ungrounded.

The only way to examine this problem definitely would be a prospective randomized control trial. This would be the one way to remove bias from the observations but it could probably never be done. It would require about 30,000 VDU-trained operators who would become pregnant and allow themselves to be randomly allocated to using or not using VDU equipment in the first twelve weeks of pregnancy. Their offspring would then be checked after birth for congenital abnormalities. Such an ideal is impossible.

There are other effects of using VDUs due to job stress and

the posture the woman has to adopt to use the unit. Eyestrain, neck ache and wrist problems do arise but these are related to the problems of prolonged sitting, possibly poor posture, and peering at the VDU screen in poor lighting conditions. None of these seem to affect the outcome of pregnancy but they are factors which could be put right very simply by proper office management.

The current state of the use of VDUs in pregnancy is best summed up in an article in the *British Journal of Obstetrics and Gynaecology* in 1988 which said: 'At present it seems reasonable to conclude that pregnancy will not be harmed by using a VDU. Statements to the contrary are not soundly based.'

Case Study

Mrs F E came to the prepregnancy clinic concerned about her work. For the last four years she had used a VDU and had acquired skills in this which led to an increased salary. She wanted to get pregnant but had many worries about the VDU. She had been told by other VDU workers that VDUs caused an increase in miscarriages and baby abnormalities.

We discussed the matter fully with her, pointing out the facts and answering her questions. She was mostly concerned about the X-rays which she thought the machines emitted. We were able to reassure her wholeheartedly on this score, for no X-radiation comes from a VDU.

She understood that she had been misled and went away with her husband to consider pregnancy. Mrs F E attended our hospital during antenatal care and was quite happy to work on her VDU apart from the problems of shoulder and wrist fatigue in pregnancy. She was safely delivered of a normal 3.5 kg (7 lb 12 oz) boy.

CHEMICAL PROBLEMS

Many chemicals have been blamed at some time for affecting the early embryo. Some of these reports again relate to small numbers of cases and such scares are easy to start but hard to rebut. The first reports become big news so there are newspaper headlines about women working in a certain factory and using certain chemicals having a higher rate of miscarriage, preterm labour or congenital abnormalities or, worse, some combination of the three. When, two or three years later, the Health and Safety Executive have investigated these claims and found that they are only chance phenomena, the facts very rarely get into the newspapers. To accuse is big news, to rebut is not.

Case Study

Miss K M was working in an agricultural research laboratory on insecticides and fungicides. She was hoping to marry soon and was worried about her work in relation to any future pregnancies. At the prepregnancy clinic we asked her about the specific chemicals she was using in her research. There was no easy answer in this case so we contacted the Health and Safety Executive who gave us their assessments on these substances. Whilst they could find nothing specific to show that they were hazardous, there was no research done which proved that they were safe.

Miss K M and her fiancé came to a subsequent visit and we explained all this to them. She decided not to risk the unknown and therefore left her job and took a post in a milk research laboratory in the same town.

Miss K M married, became pregnant and wrote to us after she had had twins at thirty-seven weeks with no problems. She was very happy to discuss the matter beforehand and even though we could not give a precise answer she was glad that we went into the matter to give her the details that were known at that time.

Some 25,000 individual chemicals are used in industry in the Western world and a further 2,000 new compounds are being introduced each year. It would be impossible to test all of these during pregnancy – there are just not enough scientists, laboratories, time or money. Again, even after all the testing, specific differences could still exist. Anything safe for rats, mice and many other primate animals may still be teratogenic (producing malformations in fetus) among humans. This was one of the problems with thalidomide even after it was known to produce abnormalities in human babies; when tested on many other species it had no effect and only the New Zealand white rabbit shared human vulnerability. Certain simple guidelines may be used; if a compound has a chemical formula similar to one that is known to affect the unborn child, it should not be used by women in early pregnancy. The Box below reviews the chemicals that are thought to have some effect on the human fetus. However, the list is not exhaustive, nor is it proven that these compounds would affect people in every case.

Drugs to be Avoided in Pregnancy

During the crucial days of fetal growth, in the first eight weeks of pregnancy, certain drugs taken by the mother can have a catastrophic effect on development. These drugs are few in number but if a woman is on any of them she should consult her doctor immediately to see whether they should be stopped.

Probably the only drugs proven to affect the fetus are thalidomide, the radioactive isotope drugs used for endocrine diseases, and the cytotoxic drugs used to suppress cancer. Thalidomide should never be used in women of the pregnancy age group, for it can cause damage to the fetal limbs. The other two groups of drugs should probably not be given and pregnancy should not be advised at any time when they are in use.

(Drugs to be Avoided in Pregnancy cont.)

There are other drugs which may have an effect on the embryo but are not as specific as the first three groups. These include the anticonvulsants taken by epileptics, warfarin used for anticoagulation, alcohol in large doses and the live vaccines that may be given to the mother to inoculate her against infectious diseases.

Another group of drugs is less likely to be harmful but reports of problems have been received. These include quinine and chloroquine, used in the prevention and treatment of malaria, and the hormones oestrogen and progesterone. These steroids are present in the combined oral contraceptive pill but their dose is very small and most women who continue inadvertently taking the pill after they are pregnant cause no harm. The trimethoprim group of sulphonamides are best avoided, for they may affect the metabolism of folic acid. Likewise, amphetamines and some diuretics should also be avoided.

This list is not exhaustive but any woman taking one or more of the drugs mentioned here should either avoid pregnancy or consult her doctor about the specific condition for which she is taking the drugs and whether they need be taken in relation to her forthcoming pregnancy.

If a woman is worried about toxic chemicals or irradiation at work, the wisest thing to do (before she is pregnant) is to consult the Health and Safety Officer at work, if the company for whom she works is big enough to have one. In their absence, the trade union officials are usually helpful. Even if the woman does not belong to a trade union, they would still assist her in this matter. If there are no such persons in her firm, she could write to the Manufacturing, Science and Finance Union, a trade union which takes a particular interest in this subject and one which has acquired a lot of relevant information. If this is not possible, she can contact the Health and Safety Executive in London (see Useful Addresses).

If you think you are working with a particular toxic hazard, you should talk about this to your employer before starting pregnancy. There are usually specific codes of practice which safeguard pregnant women and their unborn children and you could well be offered alternative work. This work should be of the same type as you are used to doing and there should be no loss of payment or benefits.

It is not enough to rely upon the usual health protection measures of screening and monitoring in the workplace. In many instances we do not know what levels of toxic substance are safe and it is best to assume that none of them are. In consequence, they should all be avoided for some weeks before the pregnancy starts. It is probable that the growing embryo is more vulnerable than the adult to these agents. Adult occupational exposure limits are based upon the currently available medical evidence.

Whilst planning before pregnancy, you should also take into account the effects of toxic substances on your new baby after birth. Breastfeeding can go on for many months after the woman returns to work and the child can receive the toxins through the breast milk. This is a less well-understood subject but generally any toxic substance that is fat-soluble can potentially go through the milk very readily. Before pregnancy has started you should therefore consult with management, the appropriate trade unions or the Health and Safety Officer.

BIOLOGICAL HAZARDS

In the workplace biological hazards involve increased risk from bacterial and viral infections which might affect the growing child. Those who work in biological laboratories are paradoxically probably the best protected, for regulations lay down very stringent protective measures. Other women working away from laboratories are often at more risk.

German measles (or rubella), if contracted in the first eight weeks of gestation, can cause abnormalities of the heart, brain or alimentary tract in the unborn child. If an infection attacks the mother later in her pregnancy the child may suffer from a chronic Rubella Syndrome with poor growth and deafness.

Teachers of small children are particularly at risk from such an infection for childhood is the most common time for rubella infections. All teachers should be checked at the beginning of their post by a simple blood test to see if rubella antibodies are present. If they are present in reasonable amounts that woman is safe in the face of infection. If the rubella antibody levels are not high enough that teacher is at risk and should be offered an inoculation of rubella antibodies to stimulate resistance.

Case Study

Mrs S L came to see us at the prepregnancy clinic because she was worried about the possibility of German measles affecting a future pregnancy. She had a neighbour who, having contracted German measles during her pregnancy, had a child who was mentally retarded and suffered from eye problems. The concern was particularly pressing for Mrs S L taught at a primary school where she was in close contact with a large number of children; if a rubella outbreak occurred in her town she would undoubtedly be in the front line.

We took a blood sample and checked her rubella antibody levels. They were negative, implying that Mrs S L had never had German measles and so had built up no antibodies to the rubella virus. In consequence, we recommended she go to her General Practitioner for inoculation and this was done. We added that Mrs S L would be wise to use oral contraception for the three months while the rubella antigen worked and this she did. Six months later, she had a substantial level of antibodies to German measles and so was happy when she became pregnant about a year after her first visit to the prepregnancy clinic.

Pregnancy progressed uneventfully. Mrs S L was delivered safely and wrote to us after the delivery, telling us of the happy event. She also mentioned that she had personally made sure that all the other teachers in her school were tested in the same way. Thus she spread the word about preventive medicine in her own community.

Non-Specific Hazards

As well as the toxic effects, there are various physiological changes that occur in pregnancy that might make work disadvantageous for the growing baby.

When any muscle action takes place, there is an increase in the output of blood from the heart. This provides the muscles with more blood, allowing them to extract oxygen and continue their work more efficiently. This process is partly achieved by shutting down the blood supply to certain less essential areas at the time of exercise; these include the kidneys, the intestines and, in extremely hard work, the uterus. Hence, during strenuous exercise, the blood supply to the leg and back muscles can go up as much as twenty times while that to the uterus may be halved. This is probably not relevant in most work for these figures refer to strenuous exercise which few women do for more than a short time. However, it might be important in bouts of hard physical work, particularly if these are repeated frequently or are prolonged, as in agricultural work.

Other effects of hard physical work are an increase in the acidity of the blood, an increase in temperature and more sweating. Individually and collectively, these factors can affect development and growth of the fetus, particularly in early pregnancy when cell changes are vital. (These problems are considered in detail in Chapter 11.)

STRESS

Many working women seeking prepregnancy care wonder about the effects of stress. It is hard to measure these precisely but the metabolic products associated with stress (the catecholamines) are increased during both work and pregnancy. In research with other species of primates, it can be shown that stress, at a sufficient level to produce agitation in the pregnant animal, causes reduction in oxygenation of the fetus. This is even more acute if the fetus is compromised already by raised blood pressure. Most work does not stress a woman mentally and if she is working within her own limits then it probably has no effect upon the fetus. However, extremely stressful work might have an effect (see Chapter 11).

CHRONIC EFFECTS OF WORK

Perhaps the major advice given at the prepregnancy clinic about work during pregnancy should not relate to the acute effects of physical exercise but the longer-term effects of fatigue. This has been investigated well in Lyons by Irène Mamelle and her colleagues who have shown the effects of fatigue on pregnancy. They have examined people working in various industrial and agricultural jobs, comparing them with those working in offices and shops.

Mme Mamelle has derived a fatigue index based upon the repetitive nature of the work, the physical effort required, the boredom resulting from work requiring little attention, the effect of having to remain standing and of working with background noise. With an increase in these various factors in a cluster of poor working conditions, there was an increase in the proportion of preterm deliveries, that is of women delivering spontaneously before the thirty-seventh week of pregnancy. These naturally resulted in smaller babies who had a higher rate of problems.

If you are going to work outside the home in pregnancy, if your partner does not already help, try to persuade him to change his habits. He may wish to help with the cooking, particularly since you are likely to come home tired at the end of the day. To have someone to prepare the supper would be a great advantage in early pregnancy when you may be feeling sick. No one learns to cook at a moment's notice so practice may be needed in the prepregnancy era. Try to get some help with the housework. The house need not be quite so spick and span during pregnancy and if you are going to work out of the house most housework will have to be done at weekends. Again, your partner might be able to share this with you. All this is best discussed before pregnancy begins.

Conclusions

The whole subject of work and pregnancy is a complex one which cannot be directed only at the job itself. The characteristics of a woman who goes out to work may often be different from those who wish to stay at home, and there are many factors – such as health, education and readiness to accept antenatal care – which could all have an effect.

The links between a woman's work and the outcome of her pregnancy are difficult to establish. In general, if a woman is doing a job which involves certain physical or chemical toxic agents, she should consult with her employers and Health and Safety Officers very carefully before considering a pregnancy. In such cases it may be wise to consider changing jobs before starting a pregnancy, for these noxious influences may adversely affect the developing embryo in the very early days of pregnancy.

The majority of women, whose employment does not involve such chemical or physical agents, would still be well-advised to consider the influence of their work in the forthcoming pregnancy. If the work is in a fairly harmonious environment and if the travel involved is not too stressful, they may in general continue throughout pregnancy. The date of stopping can be decided based on the woman's own feelings after the thirtieth week of pregnancy. If the job is a tough one, involving long hours in boring or arduous working conditions, there may be an association with risks of having an earlier delivery and a smaller baby. If you have had a preterm delivery before, you may well consider not working after mid-pregnancy or, if economics demand, trying to get work in another area. Unemployment in Britain makes this difficult at the moment but still, thinking of one's future child, it may be worth making the effort to try and find a post that allows a different work pattern.

If your job is not a high risk category you should continue working as long as you wish to. Special cases are those who already have problems or have had them in past pregnancies; such women must consider changing their work patterns. However, most working women manage a job, a partner and a baby as well as working in their home.

EIGHT

Nutrition

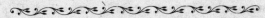

I shall be very brief in laying down this ...
and not tire your patience with the tale of a
cock and a bull; therefore consider that by
a temperate diet I intend that such an exact
quantity of meat and drink should be taken
into the stomach as the stomach is well able to
concoct and digest perfectly, which sufficeth
the due nourishment of the body.

Culpeper

In many senses we are what we eat. The food that we take in and the fluid that we drink make up body tissues which grow and sustain us through the whole of adult life. If we eat a poor diet we are liable to be thinner, even to the point of malnutrition. If food is essential, we must also accept that the unborn child is composed of that which the mother eats. Taken to an extreme, you might consider that the child depends upon the mother's appetite. This idea has given rise to folk lore and myth that says a pregnant mother should eat for two, for she needs more to sustain her growing child in the uterus. This myth is commonly perpetuated by relatives who often compete to feed up the pregnant woman. However, a woman may weigh 60 kg (9 st 5 lb) at the beginning of pregnancy and produce a baby weighing 3 kg (6 lb 9 oz). Indeed, she may eat a great deal during pregnancy, so that her weight goes up to 80 kg (12 st 8 lb) and still produce a 3 kg baby. Similarly, even if a woman eats little and increases only to 62kg (9 st 12 lb) she can produce a 3 kg baby.

It is only at the extremes of malnutrition that the birth weight of newborn children is affected. The last time this happened in the Western world was in Holland in the winter of 1944/45 when the Allies advanced inland and Holland was cut off from the rest of occupied Europe. The Germans had little food for themselves and even less for their captive civilian population. In consequence, women living under those conditions were starving and their babies were smaller.

The famine lasted from the autumn of 1944 until May 1945. Those who were already pregnant, and who gave birth in

January or February 1945, only suffered starvation for the last few months of pregnancy; they produced normal children who were only slightly lighter than expected birth weights. However, those who conceived during the time of the famine, and delivered when reasonable food supplies had got through to them in the summer and autumn of 1945, had a much higher number of miscarriages and small-for-dates babies; the number of babies who died at birth also increased. Those women who had not achieved pregnancy by the time the famine started often did not ovulate and so did not become pregnant. When they did ovulate at the end of the famine they also suffered miscarriages, small-for-dates babies and a greater number of babies dying at birth.

This emphasizes the need for prepregnancy dietary care in an extreme fashion. Fortunately the Western world has not seen a famine like this since. In other parts of the world famines occur but rarely do they start and finish with such abruptness that observations can be made, as happened during the hungry winter in Holland.

Good nutrition before pregnancy is one of the major factors in helping to produce a healthy baby. There are naturally many other factors but we have less control over these; it therefore seems sensible to look at some features which we can control. When food is taken into the body some of it is used immediately for energy or building up tissues. The rest is put into reserve and the unborn child often draws on these reserves in early pregnancy.

What Does Food Do?

In most parts of the more affluent Western world, eating is a habit. We have breakfast, lunch (or dinner), dinner (or tea or supper), each day and tend to sit down at a table to eat at those times. The quantity that we eat varies enormously according to that which we can afford and our personal preferences. We tend to eat those foods that we enjoy and those that satisfy our appetite. Appetite is the differential desire for certain foods and lack of interest in others. In this we are all built differently but appetite generally includes most edible things and excludes things that are tasteless or taste nasty.

When we take in food, we chew it to break it into a pulp which can then be swallowed. In the stomach it is subjected to acid juices which remove many harmful bacteria and help to start the digestive process by breaking down some of the larger food molecules. The semi-liquid food then passes on to the intestines where further digestion takes place. Constituents of the food are broken down into smaller molecules which are absorbed into the bloodstream through the wall of the intestine. What is left passes on to the large intestine; water is extracted from it and the residue is passed out through the anus in the form of stools. This residue contains a great deal of fibre, the bulk of the food. In addition, bile is actively secreted from the liver; the bile consists of breakdown products and many byproducts of drugs taken by mouth which are thereby passed out of the body in the stools.

All the food that we eat can be divided into several groups. These are: carbohydrates (energy-giving foods); proteins (tissue-balancing foods); fats (solvent and appetite foods); vitamins (catalysts for all body processes); minerals (minute but essential components of tissues); fibre (unabsorbable material essential for the passage of food through the alimentary tract); and water (present in all food and essential for maintaining the shape and size of all cells).

Some understanding of these various groups of foodstuffs is necessary to unravel the tangled skein of advice that is given to people, pregnant or prepregnant, about nutrition.

Carbohydrates
These energy-giving foods range from simple sugars to the more complex starches and celluloses. Glucose and fructose are natural sugars found in many fruits and in honey. Glucose

is the sugar made when starches are digested in the body. These sugars all dissolve easily in water and have a sweet taste. The celluloses are the more complex, very big molecules found abundantly in the plant kingdom. These are taken into the body and broken down by digestion into glucose. The sugars are carried in the blood to muscles where they are broken down to give energy, thus enabling the muscles to work. The reserve stores of carbohydrates are mainly in the form of glycogen, a complex molecule manufactured in the liver. Some organs, such as the brain, cannot store glycogen and therefore have very small reserves of energy-producing substances.

Proteins

Proteins are found in all living cells and provide the basic structure of all tissues. They are made up of complex arrangements of amino acids. Vegetarian animals, such as cows, get their proteins by eating plants, whilst carnivorous creatures obtain their proteins from the flesh of other animals. Omnivores, like humans, get protein from both sources although preference may lead some individuals more to a vegetable than an animal source.

When proteins are eaten, they are broken down by digestion into the basic amino acids and these are carried in the blood to various parts of the body. They combine again to form proteins in the cells by building up tissues. Hence, more proteins are required at a time of growth, like pregnancy, than at other times.

Plant foods which contain large proportions of protein include many of the bean family, such as soya and peanuts. Amongst animal foods, eggs, cheese and meat are rich in protein.

To some extent, amino acids can be reconstituted in the body so one can be transformed into another. However there are fifteen essential amino acids which cannot be so constructed and have to be taken in direct from food. Most of these occur in both plants and animals but two of them are in animal sources only. Hence, a vegetarian may need assistance with these essential amino acids. If the vegetarian diet includes milk and cheese, this provides a full range of amino acids and such a woman need not be concerned that she is not going to provide enough amino acids for her child. If, however, she is a vegan and takes no animal produce at all, in the prepregnancy period and during pregnancy itself she would be wise to adapt her diet, with advice from her doctor, to include some primary amino acids for the sake of her baby.

Fats

These are found in both animals and plants. Liquid fats (or oils) may occur in both but animal fats are usually solid, although at body temperature they may appear liquid; fats do not dissolve in water. They provide energy and also act as the intermediary substance in the cell walls through which essential molecules can be transported from one cell to another.

Fats are made up of glycerine and a variety of fatty acids (complex organic molecules). When taken into the body they are broken down by digestion so that the fatty acids are absorbed. Some are immediately burnt up to provide energy and others are stored; fat stores are commonly found under the skin where they also give us a layer of insulation against loss of heat from the body.

In pregnancy, fatty acids do not usually cross from the mother to the fetus. Instead, fats are made in the fetus itself from basic organic substances, particularly in the latter part of pregnancy.

Vitamins

Vitamins are chemical compounds required to catalyse reactions in the body. Minute amounts are needed but without them the reaction cannot take place. They might be compared to the detonators needed to make an explosive substance start firing.

A loose group of compounds, vitamins bear no relation to each other, apart from their catalytic mechanisms. They were first discovered in 1910, and the alphabetical letters allocated to them simply signify the order in which they were found; there is no nutritional logic or reason in their allocation.

Vitamins are found in association with various foods. So little is required of any individual vitamin, even in the pregnancy stage, that any woman in the Western world who eats a reasonably mixed diet is getting ample amounts of vitamins. No benefit is gained from taking any extra vitamins on top of an adequate diet for they are not absorbed into the body; they pass straight through into the lavatory pan. Vitamin supplements are quite unnecessary for people on ordinary mixed diets in the United Kingdom. Furthermore, it can be dangerous to take an excess of certain vitamins; hypervitaminosis – the condition of poisoning from too much of any given vitamin – exists for all the known vitamins.

If a woman lives on a diet composed of only a few food substances, then she is likely to be short of certain vitamins that are associated with the missing foods in the diet. Perhaps the most common vitamin deficiencies are scurvy, caused by absence of vitamin C which occurs in fresh fruit, and beriberi, due to absence of vitamin B found in cereals. These are exceedingly rare in the United Kingdom and represent the extremes of malnutrition.

Some deficiencies have been associated with specific changes in the unborn child. However, these reports are often not fully understood by the newspapers that report them, for many of them are biased towards the making of a news story rather than honest reporting. A good example is the association of vitamin deficiency with spina bifida which is dealt with later in this chapter. First reports showed a loose association between the two but these results were exaggerated by those who wished to promote the use of vitamins for a variety of reasons. Later studies, which showed that these associations may have been due to chance, have been nothing like so well reported.

VITAMIN A

This is originally made in rapidly growing plants and taken into the body when animals eat them. The vitamin is stored in the fat of animals or fish and thus arrives in the human diet. It has an effect on eyesight, and the health of skin, teeth and bones. Vitamin A is present in large quantities in milk, eggs and liver, as well as most vegetables, particularly lettuce, carrots and turnips.

VITAMIN B

The B group is a loose complex of vitamins of which there are at least six members. The lack of vitamin B1 leads to beriberi in which the nerves become inflamed, causing paralysis of the limbs. Vitamin B1 cannot be stored in the body and so it needs to be replaced constantly. It is found in fresh fruits, cereals and enriched flour. Vitamin B2 is associated with the orderly division of cells in growth and is generally found in green leafy vegetables, milk and liver.

VITAMIN C

This vitamin is found in fresh citrus fruits and it too cannot be stored for any length of time. It is replaced by a daily intake of citrus fruits or their products (oranges, lemons or grapefruit).

VITAMIN D

Fish oils (cod liver oil), liver and egg yolks are all rich in vitamin D. It can also be made by humans from the action of sunlight on the skin. In consequence, deficiency is rare in warmer countries but may occur in parts of the temperate Western world, particularly among people who cover themselves up and do not allow the sun to reach their skin, as do many Islamic women. This vitamin is concerned with the growth of bones.

VITAMIN E

Vitamin E is often associated with reproduction. It is found in most foods and is stored for a long time in the body so people rarely need any extra sources of this vitamin.

VITAMIN K

This is an essential catalyst in the clotting mechanisms of the blood. It is found in dark green leaf plants, such as spinach, cabbage and cauliflower, and from animal sources in liver. Many newborn babies are short of vitamin K, as metabolism of this particular vitamin is often poor in the newborn liver. In hospitals vitamin K is given by drops or injection at birth.

Minerals

The three major constituents of food – carbohydrate, protein and fat – are all used to provide energy and build tissue. Minerals are in a different class. They are needed in minute quantities, mostly to provide essential chemical links in the enzymes which run the body. These chemical messengers link all our physical and mental processes; every time we think, move, breathe or digest food, we need enzymes to help the process. Minerals provide minute but essential parts of the enzymes which make them act. Although we require very small amounts, minerals are a vital part of our dietary intake.

Some minerals are needed to replace normal intra- and extra-cellular enzymes, and are taken in quantities of less than 10 mg a day (the amount that would appear on the head of a pin). These are calcium, phosphorus, magnesium, sodium, potassium and chloride. All these are excreted from the body in the urine and therefore have to be replaced. Even smaller amounts of certain essential trace elements are required. These are zinc, copper, iodine, fluorine, manganese and chromium.

Most minerals can be obtained from natural foods. If doctors think you are not getting enough from your own food they would recommend taking a mineral supplement, but this is very unusual. The only mineral supplement that is required in pregnancy is iron and this will be discussed later on.

Only in extreme cases can one determine if a woman is short of minerals by taking a sample of blood, hair, sweat or saliva. If the diet is sufficient to satisfy her energy needs and protein requirements, she will usually have more than enough of all the minerals she requires as well as most of the vitamins, so no further supplements are required.

Fibre

We do not absorb all that we eat. Much vegetable material is in the form of plant cellulose which we cannot digest. In this we differ from herbivores, such as rabbits, who obtain much of their energy by breaking cellulose down into sugars. The fibre provides the roughage and is necessary to act as carrier of all essential foods through the intestines. Without it, transport would soon stop and nutrients would no longer be absorbed from the various parts of the intestinal tract.

Fibre has one essential function in nutrition and that is water storage. It holds water in amongst its cellular matter until the food products reach the large intestine. There, in the lower reaches of that long organ, water is reabsorbed into the body from the food matter; thus are formed the firmer stools which are passed periodically from the rectum. In the human species stools are not stored in the anal canal or rectum itself but a little higher up in the sigmoid colon.

Fibre is obtained mainly from vegetable sources. Most vegetables, particularly cereals and root vegetables, contain it. Good portions of these taken as part of the diet will provide quite enough fibre to keep you adequately maintained. A sure sign of decreased fibre is constipation when the stools become hard pellets and are not easy to pass. This can often be cured by taking adequate fibre in order to carry more water down to the lower end of the intestinal tract.

Water

Water is essential for all life and it is the main constituent of the human body. As much as 70 to 80% of the body consists of water and even such apparently solid tissues as bone contain large quantities of it. All cells contain water; the minerals are dissolved and the larger protein molecules held in suspension in cell water. The nucleus of the cells is held in this water environment and exchange takes place by movement of molecules through the water of the cell. Thus the molecules move across the membrane and into the fluid outside the cell, communicating with the bloodstream.

All foods, even dry bread, contain water, though some foods obviously contain more than others. In addition to the food we eat, we drink water in all the beverages we take. It is essential to have plenty of water; within reason it is hard to overdo the water intake of a healthy body, for the kidney will regulate the amount of water by excreting the excess in the urine. However, this does not mean that it is advisable to drink large quantities of the various beverages that are made with water, such as tea, coffee or alcohol. These may be quite safe in moderation but it should not be forgotten that they are tissue poisons if taken in large amounts.

At certain times one feels more thirsty than others. When we are warm, extra water is needed, for we lose up to 1 litre (just under 2 pints) a day through the skin when we sweat moderately. Certain salty foods also make us thirsty; we should take in more water to hold this salt in solution in the body, not allowing a rise in the concentration of these salts in the body fluids.

Eating to Feed the Baby

These are the essential nutrients which are required in various proportions in prepregnancy and during pregnancy. Having been taken in, they are absorbed in a simplified form through the intestine. Some are then stored in parts of the body and they circulate in the blood according to the concentration of existing nutrients.

The growing embryo extracts nutrients from the mother's blood in various ways according to the stage of gestation. At first, the fertilized egg in its early cellular stage passes slowly down the Fallopian tube (as described in Chapter 2). At this point, all nutrients must be obtained from the fluids excreted by the cells which line the Fallopian tube. This fluid is the only source of food for the early embryo at a time when it is actively dividing and using up energy sources very rapidly.

By day eight or nine, the developing egg, now known as the blastocyst, has passed into the uterus. While resting on the lining of the uterus it is dependent upon endometrial fluids to provide the nutrients and to remove the waste products from the surface of the mass of cells. The blastocyst now implants, sinking into the uterine lining, disorganizing maternal tissues as it does so. It is thus surrounded by the mother's blood, from which it extracts nutrients as well as oxygen, disposing of carbon dioxide and other waste products directly back into the mother's blood.

Soon growth of the blastocyst prevents the innermost cells from obtaining their nutrients by simple diffusion and a blood supply is needed; this starts on about day twenty-two of development (as described in Chapter 2). The surface of the blastocyst is covered with many finger-like protrusions which enlarge the area at which exchange can take place. As the growing embryo develops and organs are laid down in the following weeks the surface exchange area shrinks back to one-fifth of the surface of the uterine lining and takes on a disc-like form; this is the placenta. The placenta is in direct relationship with maternal blood and all exchange now occurs across the placental wall for the rest of pregnancy.

The placenta is arranged so as to provide an enormous surface area with a very thin membrane just separating the maternal blood from the fetal blood. The maternal blood arrives at the placental bed from about 200 arteries which are branches of the main artery to the uterus. These jet the mother's blood under moderate pressure into a pool into which dips the fetal placenta; the exchange area is greatly magnified by numerous finger-like protrusions which make the effective surface area of the placenta about the size of a tennis court. Exchange can therefore take place fairly easily between the maternal blood and fetal circulation across a single layer of cells.

Different nutrients enter the fetus in different ways. The carbohydrates pass entirely as sugars, small molecules which diffuse across the membrane easily. The higher concentration of sugars found in the mother's blood eases the passage by diffusion across to the fetal blood where there are lower concentrations. In this way the sugars pass into the fetal blood by a simple process of osmosis*.

The proteins pass entirely as amino acids* which cross the placenta against a concentration gradient, thus accumulating amino acids in the fetus at a higher level than in the mother. These have different methods of crossing the placenta depending on their chemical structure. This starts with absorption from the maternal blood onto the surface of the cells of the placental membrane. Active transport across the cell wall itself is followed by another active process across the second membrane on the fetal side of the cellular barrier. Active transport requires energy which is provided by carbohydrates and this allows amino acids to accumulate in the fetus.

As has been previously explained, fats do not transfer across the placenta and the fat laid down in the fetus is made in the fetus itself from other chemical constituents.

Vitamins are transferred to the fetus passively depending upon their solubility. The fat-soluble vitamins (A and D) are diffused across the fat supplements in the walls of the cells separating the maternal and fetal circulations. This is an easy process from the higher concentrations of vitamins in the mother's blood to lower vitamin concentrations in the fetus. The water-soluble vitamins (B, C and E) are actively transported with water but then convert into non-transportable forms. Hence, fetal levels of most vitamins are higher than those of the mother so that a fetus would respond quicker to a high vitamin level than would the mother. This is important when unnecessary extra vitamins are given to women in pregnancy.

Water passes across to the unborn child according to the concentrations of molecules on either side of the feto-maternal membranes. Generally there is a flux into the fetus but this is not the only passage for the fetal needs of water. In addition, the fetus swallows some of the amniotic fluid which surrounds him like a swimming pool inside the mother's uterus, and this is absorbed by the intestine. He further secretes fluid by means of the not-very-efficient fetal kidneys back into that swimming pool. The amniotic fluid communicates with the maternal bloodstream through all the membranes surrounding the growing pregnancy and this is another variable of water excretion. Generally there is enough fluid in the amniotic pool to protect the baby from mechanical buffeting and temperature changes but occasionally this becomes abnormally small (oligohydramnios) or abnormally great (polyhydramnios).

Determining Nutrient Needs

If a woman is eating a normal mixed diet before pregnancy she is undoubtedly taking enough of the basic nutrients to keep her and her growing child healthy through pregnancy. Should she have an abnormal diet or should her absorption be poor, then there may be a reason to supplement her diet. This will be discussed shortly.

Total malnutrition is rare except under extreme circumstances, such as those already described in Holland during the Second World War. More commonly there is one component of the diet which becomes lacking, particularly if there is a poor income and the woman has to depend upon cheaper foods to stave off hunger. Often, other children in the household will get the best of the food and the working mother will take the less protein-rich items. Further, when meals are prepared in haste, convenience foods may be used in preference to those that contain more balanced quantities of proteins, vitamins and minerals. These deficiencies are all difficult to prove and the changes produced are subtle.

Is there any way of telling when a diet is short of any vital constituents? Classically, a scientist could find out what is being taken in by obtaining a sample of the diet and analysing its various constituents. This is not easy, for the analysis is not a simple one. It can be done for special studies but it is time-consuming and difficult to apply in practice. A slightly less precise method would be to consult a dietitian who would discuss the diet actually taken. She would want a diary filled in for a week or two with the foods taken and their estimated quantity. She could then consult sources which give the constituents of the various foods eaten and so accumulate a list of the component parts of the diet. She might then be able to advise on gross deficiencies of certain elements. Both these methods have been used in assessment of pregnant and prepregnant women using large numbers of women in special surveys but they are difficult to apply to the individual.

The clinical signs of vitamin and mineral deficiency come very late and are gross end points in the process of deficiency. By the time anyone develops pellagra or scurvy, the deficiency of vitamin B or C would have been going on for a long time and have reached a very severe level. One therefore has to rely on general advice about a healthy diet.

In recent years it has become fashionable to measure levels of certain vitamins or minerals in various body tissues, such as the blood, urine, saliva or hair. Because numbers are produced, this has the air of scientific measurement, and gives the impression of being an acceptable and reliable method. However, none of these tissues are capable of providing such information. Blood is a transport medium carrying nutrients and other substances from one part of the body to the other. It merely reflects what is put into it and taken out of it at any given time and not the total state of the body. Further, in the blood certain substances are bound to protein molecules and therefore, though they would appear on the analysis, they are not available for use in the body. Such bindings would greatly affect the useful concentrations of substances in the blood.

The urine contains the end products of metabolism. Excretion patterns alter enormously during the day and so the actual concentration in the urine is not a precise measure of what is going on inside the body. Similarly, measurement of compounds in saliva might seem to be a potential method of assessing one aspect of the body's metabolism although it is not used very much. In the saliva, substances are excreted from the body either by spitting or by swallowing, but the substances are changed by the acid of the stomach.

The hair is a dumping ground into which products are unloaded via the hair follicles of the scalp. Levels of minerals there reflect the concentration in the blood and the transfer processes that occurred some weeks or months earlier. Hair growth can be fairly easily estimated and so, theoretically, one can tell from the length of hair approximately when the piece cut off was actually in the follicles. However the variations of deposition are enormous in hair follicles and produce far too wide a range of results to be really useful.

The *Observer* newspaper of Sunday, 22 May 1988, reported a simple test when one of the women journalists took a sample of hair from her head and divided it into two even parts. These were enclosed in envelopes and labelled with two different names. The two envelopes were sent to the same laboratory and were analysed for certain elements. The results are summarized in the table below.

Results of Hair Analysis

	Hair A mg/kg	Hair B mg/kg
Calcium	407	269
Magnesium	35	26
Phosphorus	117	126
Sodium	102	72
Potassium	54	22
Iron	29	32
Copper	16	23
Zinc	102	196
Chromium	0.68	0.71
Manganese	0.16	0.8
Selenium	1.6	1.6
Nickel	0.5	0.77
Cobalt	0.13	0.09

The laboratory reported that one of the envelopes contained the hair of someone who was deficient in magnesium, sodium, potassium, manganese and cobalt while the other apparently had a zinc deficiency. The hairs sent were cut at the same distance from the scalp in each case and so it was not a question of the deposition of one month being different from another.

The hair results are perhaps an extreme case but any blood level would show great variations of a given dietary substance throughout the day, with the highest level being at least twice that of the lowest. Which should be taken as normal? Biochemical measuring methods have now outstripped our understanding of dietary matters. In many cases a gullible public is therefore exposed to a new dietary supplement philosophy which is mostly untested.

In pregnancy a woman needs about 400 kilo-calories a day in addition to her normal energy requirements. About half of this will be provided by the altered efficiency of energy utilization inside the body. Hence, between 200 and 300 extra kilo-calories a day need to be consumed. If this were taken in the form of a mixed diet in the United Kingdom it would more than provide the extra 10 g of protein required each day, and would give most of the vitamins and all the minerals that are needed. A woman should therefore eat her own mixed diet to her own appetite within the limits of acceptable weight gain. According to medical physiologists, women following such a regimen would probably require no supplements at all.

The whole problem of dietary intake in and out of pregnancy is compounded by the various national and international bodies who lay down daily requirements for individuals. These requirements are perhaps important in planning at a national level but are of less use for the individual. They are designed to cover all possible contingencies and thus look at the worst state.

Further, if one compares the recommended daily allowance of many of the nutrients, there is an enormous variation from one country to another. For example folate, the vitamin B that is needed for growth, is probably utilized at a rate of about 180 micrograms per day in the middle of pregnancy. The Canadian recommended daily requirement is 50, while in New Zealand it is 300 micrograms. Similarly, calcium is either under-represented in Indonesia which suggests 100 micrograms or grossly over-represented in Argentina where 400 micrograms a day are recommended. Likewise with zinc, a contentious metal in dietary terms, the range of recommended daily intake shows a variation four times the utilized dose.

On the whole, many of these diet requirements are best ignored by the individual. The special cases are dealt with later; if you think you have a problem in your diet or the absorption of diet, ask your obstetrician or prepregnancy counsellor who will give you individual advice on this. In most cases, a rea-sonable mixed diet will give all a woman needs in pregnancy or prepregnancy.

The Healthy Diet

Having decided that the ordinary mixed diet is going to provide most of what is required in prepregnancy, how may a woman obtain this? Very few people go out shopping with lists of nutrients in mind. They buy food rather than nutrients. This can be translated very simply by ensuring that you buy food from various groups. For instance, one could divide ordinary foods into protein providers, calorie providers, fibre providers and fresh fruits.

The protein providers may be either meat, fish, eggs, pulses or seeds. Meats do not have to be the most expensive cuts of fillet steak. Stewing steaks are just as nutritious, and the organ meats of liver, kidneys and heart are just as tasty. These last contain many vitamins and minerals and, if it is to your taste, fried liver and onions once a week or a stuffed lamb's heart is a great delicacy and provides excellent nutrition. Fish is often cheaper than meat and is more than just a vehicle for a sauce. Fresh fish has excellent flavours in its own right, and has become more widely available in the United Kingdom. Oily fish

– herrings, mackerels and sardines – contain many nutrients, particularly the fat-soluble vitamins. Finally, the various beans now sold through health food shops and supermarkets are an excellent source of plant proteins and are very cheap.

The calorie providers include starches, sugars and fats. Starches come in flour and, although the sliced white loaf still dominates the market, wholemeal bread contains more vitamins and minerals as well as calories. The root vegetables also provide starches, whilst rice and pasta are good wholesome foods for calorie provision. These are all better than the sweet sugars which occur in biscuits and of course in sugar itself. Whilst such sugars give some energy, much of this goes towards weight increase without helping particularly in nutrition. Many people have a sweet tooth and they should try to satisfy this with natural sugars (honey and fruits) rather than with sugar from a packet. In the Western world many calories are provided by fat. The trouble is that fat also increases weight. In addition, it contains cholesterol and low density lipoproteins which can lead to problems of clotting in blood vessels. Although it is very well flavoured and appetizing, fat should therefore be restricted in a diet.

Fibre comes from fruit and vegetables, particularly the very chewy ones. Another source of fibre is the cereals and brans eaten for breakfast. Most outlets now stock a wide variety of these, ranging from those based upon a whole grain to others that have many flavourings, colourings and additives (including plastic models). A swift examination of the side of the packet will give you some idea of the amount of fibre. Do not be led astray by the lists of added vitamins and minerals. As discussed earlier, these are quite unnecessary for most people and will simply be excreted.

Fresh fruit is not very expensive and is usually available all year round with worldwide marketing. Citrus fruits contain vitamin C and some natural sugars. An orange or grapefruit you can take each day as part of a healthy diet and if these are not acceptable lemon juice can usually be added to drink or food. Apples and pears provide roughage with their fibre as well as natural sugars. Strawberries, raspberries and blackberries are rich in vitamin C, whilst pineapples and dates have a high content of folate (vitamin B).

The reader may notice that milk is absent from this essential diet. Milk is a good source of calcium if you are not getting it from some other dairy product, such as cheese, or from some natural food, such as sardines or cereals containing wheatgerm. However, it also contains a lot of fat and if you drink more than 300 ml (half a pint) of milk a day, you are liable to put on detrimental fat as well as getting an excess of calcium, much of which will not be absorbed. The place of milk as a health food has been over-exaggerated and half a pint a day of whole milk is about right in the prepregnancy period, providing some cheese is also being taken.

All these foods can be obtained in various forms and the exact choice lies not just with the woman herself but also with other members of the family. However, remembering that the mother-to-be should have a portion from each of these groups of foods in the main meal each day will help in the weekly shop. Care must be taken to ensure that the modern marketing techniques do not overcome the commonsense of the woman in the prepregnancy period. Manufacturers of prepared or processed foods are now obliged to list all the ingredients on the labels, and this may help.

Try to avoid being a food faddist. If your income is low, it is important not to economize on food in the prepregnancy period. You may have to go easy on the buying of clothes or furniture but not food as this is essential for the development of your baby. If time allows, preparing fresh food rather than using pre-prepared meals will provide more nutrition. It is not only the expensive meats that are nutritious, the same applies to fish and vegetables. Many books tell you about sensible preparation for pregnancy foods and a browse around the local library shelves will be of great value at this stage.

Careless cooking habits can undo much of the good derived from careful shopping. Cookery books will advise on this but generally longer cooking of meats at a moderate temperature provides a better protein intake than short high temperature cooking. Basting with the meat's own fat protects it from direct heat. Poaching or baking fish is better than grilling or barbecueing. When preparing vegetables, scrub them, and try to leave some of the peel on, for much of the nutrition is just under the skin. This particularly applies to baked potatoes. When preparing other vegetables do not cut them into very small portions and do not overheat them, for this renders the vitamins ineffective. Steaming may take a little longer than boiling but it leaves more nutrients in the food. Alternatively, stir-frying your vegetables quickly in a wok or shallow frying pan will seal the surface and leave the vitamins inside.

Again, an hour in the local library will provide excellent advice on these matters and thus increase both the pleasure and the nutrition of the diet that you and your partner are taking. Books are recommended at the end of this chapter.

In summary, the prepregnancy diet should help the mother-to-be prepare for her pregnancy by laying in reserves of good nutrients. This same diet will be taken during the early weeks of pregnancy to help her growing embryo develop organs and tissues properly. There is a great variation in individual needs and individual appetites. Many improvements have been made in nutrition education for pregnancy and help can be obtained from your local hospital, or the local library.

The best general advice in the prepregnancy period would be to cut down on fats, meats, sugar and salt, whilst increasing the protein from vegetables and the fibre content from cereals, wholemeal bread and fresh fruit. Following these simple guidelines, most women will be provided with a good prepregnancy diet containing all the vitamins and minerals required.

Are Supplements Required?
If a normal woman has a normal mixed diet, as described in this chapter, then no dietary supplements are likely to be required. There is no need to increase the protein but she might need to shift the balance from animal to plant proteins. Unless

she is losing weight, the calorie content is probably enough; special cases are dealt with later, but for most, the main food constituents of a balanced diet are sufficient.

A great mythology has built up around vitamins and minerals in prepregnancy and pregnancy. As has been said previously, there is probably no need to supplement these in the ordinary diet; despite this, in the United Kingdom over sixteen million pounds are spent each year on dietary supplements, mostly minerals and vitamins. Professor John Garrow, the Rank Professor of Human Nutrition at St Bartholomew's Hospital in London, explained in 1988 that at that time there was no evidence to show that many people in Britain were on inadequate diets before or during pregnancy. As he put it: 'If you are satisfying your energy requirements from ordinary food, it is quite hard to become deficient in anything. So far as minerals are concerned, I do not know of any evidence that there is any benefit to the population of taking supplements. I should be surprised if there were.'

Other eminent nutritionists make similar comments about healthy people taking vitamins. It must be remembered that the body requires very small amounts of vitamins and probably has quite enough of these in the ordinary diet. To add to these would not lead to improved nutrition; they might be absorbed and lead to a toxic level of vitamins in the blood, but in most women they would just not be absorbed from the intestine, but would pass on and end up in the stools without having any effect at all on the body. A few may be absorbed, but they will circulate round the body, not being taken up by the tissues, and be excreted in the urine. In consequence the vitamin tablets many people take in the prepregnancy period might as well be dumped straight down the lavatory or, to save money, not be bought at all.

A trace element which has been the subject of great interest recently is zinc. Elemental zinc is a very important metal, being associated with over 80 enzymes that are essential to the smooth running of the body. Deficiency has been linked with congenital abnormalities in monkeys, and in some countries low levels of zinc in the blood have been associated with a high instance of abnormalities amongst women. Similarly, there are high rates of assorted abnormalities in countries such as Iran, Egypt and India, where there is a chronic zinc deficiency in the diet. Paradoxically, taking in large amounts of zinc has also coincided with fetal loss and growth retardation in some animals. These experiments have naturally not been performed in humans. From such beginnings, the story of supplementary zinc has arisen. It has undoubtedly been fuelled by people who measure zinc in the blood or hair of women in their laboratories and then offer to sell them zinc tablets to supplement their diet.

This is a difficult area because there is no evidence that zinc deficiency is a major cause of problems in humans. Zinc levels in the blood may well be reduced in pregnancy because of the normal dilution effect that blood undergoes in pregnancy. Further, since zinc is bound to the protein albumin in the blood the amount measured by laboratory tests might not represent the amount that is actually available to be used. Having said this, it is obvious that certain minerals are required in pregnancy and zinc might well be one of them. For example, in the laboratories at St George's Hospital Medical School we have shown that the fluid secreted from the lining of the Fallopian tube to nourish the fertilized egg in the first days of life has an increased zinc content.

Zinc is so readily available in food that it is a gross exaggeration to make a scare of zinc deficiency. It is found in most meats, wholemeal bread, cheese, and in carrots and tomatoes in more than adequate amounts. Isobel Cole Hamilton, dietitian to the London Food Commission, an independent organization, said recently: 'If people were eating a healthy diet with plenty of fruit, vegetables and lean meat they would be getting all the zinc, iron, vitamins and other minerals they need without having to worry about the minute details.'

It may even be harmful to consume too much zinc, for this could prevent your body from absorbing enough calcium and iron. In 1988 the *Drug and Therapeutics Bulletin* said: 'Books distributed by health food stores suggest that many people lack zinc, and this may explain problems ranging from brittle nails to impotence. These sweeping claims are unsubstantiated.' Such books tend to mix unphysiological measurements of minerals in prepregnancy women with the potential effects of zinc deficiency on the fetus, causing a great deal of confusion. There is as yet no solid evidence that zinc deficiency exists in humans eating a mixed diet or that it has any effect in the prepregnancy period.

Myths have also grown up about the taking of iron in the prepregnancy period. According to the folk hypothesis, iron will be required in pregnancy to supply the growing baby's blood and muscles and in consequence it would be wise to build up stores before the woman gets pregnant in order to provide the baby with the iron. However, this is based on some false premises. Not all women need extra iron even in pregnancy. During the nine months of pregnancy they save much iron that is usually lost in the blood lost in menstruation each month. Further, in pregnancy absorption of iron from the intestines improves by as much as 40%. Most normal women on a normal diet therefore have enough iron in pregnancy to supply themselves and their unborn child. It is still sensible to have a haemoglobin check at a prepregnancy consultation; if anaemia is found then treatment should be given, for anyone who is anaemic requires treatment.

Very few people in the United Kingdom are anaemic (probably less than 5% of the pregnancy age group) and it is unnecessary for those who are not anaemic to increase their iron intake. Indeed, it may do harm because the presence of extra iron in the food can alter the absorption of other constituents like vitamin C from the intestine. Absorption from the intestine is a balanced and interrelated series of processes; to increase one aspect of it arbitrarily by taking a supplement could alter the usual patterns of absorption. Rather than interfering with one aspect which we think at that moment is important (perhaps because of false interpretation of data), it would be wiser to improve the woman's total nutrition in the prepregnancy period using the general measures discussed already.

A Note on Food Poisoning

Recently there has been much publicity about food poisoning, especially in relation to early pregnancy. It is important to keep this in perspective, for food poisoning is not a new condition. Bacteria exist in all the food we eat, and in many cases are important for the production of the actual flavouring of food itself, for example cheese. All the same, woman awaiting pregnancy should try to reduce the risks of encountering harmful bacteria.

In the last few years, the dangers of *Listeria* infection to the unborn child have become apparent. This organism is an inhabitant of some foods of gamey flavour – the ripe cheeses like Camembert and Brie and some pâtés – and also in cold prepared meats. Many precooked frozen meals also contain *Listeria*, as do a high proportion of chicken carcasses. The cheeses and pâtés are eaten raw; however, sensible precautions can guard a woman in immediate prepregnancy and during early pregnancy. Avoiding the uncooked products that might contain *Listeria* still leaves the hard and processed cheeses and cheese spreads to be enjoyed. Cooking the meat products at the correct temperature will give protection, but when cooking meat or heating particular precooked frozen meals, attention should be paid to the use of microwave ovens as the heating can be patchy in these. It is very important to follow the manufacturer's instructions and allow enough time for the heat to reach all parts of the food.

Not so common in the United Kingdom, but still a risk, is toxoplasmosis. This is associated with meat products, and again, proper cooking can get rid of the infective organisms. If infection were to occur very early in pregnancy it could pass to the embryo. Treatments are not very effective, so it is wise to avoid toxoplasmosis by keeping away from raw or undercooked meats, particularly in continental countries where the organism is much more common.

In the United Kingdom the producers of food and those who sell it are very careful about the standards they maintain, but one should be careful, particularly with chilled or frozen food. It would be unwise to buy any food past its sell-by date, or from a display cabinet which looks overfilled or improperly cared for. It is probably sensible not to buy cracked eggs.

Get the food home as quickly as possible and do not leave it at room temperature for long; put chilled and frozen food into the refrigerator or freezer straightaway. Remember, the fridge does not kill bacteria but simply slows down the growth of most common ones. Ensure that your refrigerator is at the ideal temperature (between 0° and 5°C). Any cooked food should be kept separate from other foods to avoid contamination; do not let meat drip onto fresh vegetables. The freezer does not kill bacteria either but only stops them multiplying. The ideal temperature will be given on the inside of the door; it should be around −18°C. Obey the instructions on food packaging and keep in the freezer for no longer than the advised storage time.

In the kitchen, cleanliness is obviously important, and you should always wash your hands before preparing food. All meat should be cooked thoroughly, particularly poultry. When food is cooked from the frozen state it is essential to ensure that it is cooked through, and poultry especially should be defrosted completely before cooking.

Recent advice from the Department of Health would indicate that raw eggs should not be eaten. For those wishing to become pregnant it is probably wise to eat eggs quite hard-boiled, with the yolk solid rather than liquid.

Recooking of food in microwave ovens needs special care. The food should *never* be reheated more than once, and then it should be very hot when served. Manufacturers' instructions will tell you how much time you need to allow for the heat to go right through the food, and these should be followed.

Salmonella and *Listeria* have held the headlines for the last few years but these are not the only bacteria which might contaminate food and lead to food poisoning. For safety for the woman in early pregnancy and during prepregnancy, these simple guidelines should be followed.

Weight

Correct body weight is the end result of adequate nutrition. During pregnancy a woman will increase her weight, most women putting on about 10 kg (22 lb). This is made up of the baby, plus placenta and amniotic fluid which also weigh several kilograms; the increased tissue laid down in the uterus and breasts and the increase in blood volume. Finally, many women put on some extra fat during pregnancy. All this is normal pregnancy gain.

Before pregnancy, weight gain is of less benefit. If somebody is underweight they may be so undernourished that they are not producing an egg each cycle. This will lead to a lack of menstruation (amenorrhoea). Such a woman would obviously need some improvement in nutrition to increase her weight, but this might not be socially acceptable. For example, dancers in the *corps de ballet* of a big company may wish to keep their sylph-like figures for dancing. This involves them in more dietary restrictions than most women would accept and is often accompanied by amenorrhoea and lack of ovulation. When their ambition to become a secondary dancer or even a prima ballerina fades, they are then able to eat a more normal diet so that menstruation and ovulation return. It is not always acceptable to advise a woman merely to eat to make her menstruate. Her work and social circumstances must be taken into consideration as well.

Even if a woman's weight loss is not so great that it causes non-ovulation, it might still be important in the prepregnancy period, for it might imply poor nutrition. It would be far better to use a balanced healthy diet to restore this woman to her normal weight rather than stuffing her like a Strasbourg goose with high calorie foods.

For many years it has been noticed that women with a low prepregnancy weight produce low birth weight babies. Weight, in relation to height, before pregnancy is a crude indicator of prepregnancy nutrition but the lower the mother's prepregnancy weight the higher the risk of having a baby of low birth weight. There is a much weaker link between low infant birth weights and maternal height than prepregnancy weight. It must be remembered that there is a time lag between a change of diet and its physiological results; in consequence, if a woman wishes to be of reasonable weight in the prepregnancy period, this may involve six to twelve months of preparation beforehand.

Margaret and Arthur Wynn examined nutrition in and around pregnancy for many years and in 1987 spoke at UNICEF, drawing attention to many studies showing how nutrition deficiencies before pregnancy affect embryonic growth at the very early egg stage. Cell division was less frequent and took more time among those who became pregnant when they were underweight. This may be due to the egg follicle* being affected even before fertilization. The cells that remain behind in the ovary after ovulation become the corpus luteum*, the organ that produces the hormone progesterone*. This hormone supports the developing embryo for the first eight to ten weeks of pregnancy. Since the corpus luteum is formed in the cells of what was the follicle before ovulation, and there is no increase in the number of cells after ovulation, the effect of prepregnancy nutrition deficiency on the follicle might affect corpus luteum production of progesterone in early pregnancy.

Japanese studies in the 1980s have shown that mice kept on a low protein diet have had, on average, ten times the number of abnormal fertilized eggs per mouse than those mice who had a standard protein prepregnancy diet. It would seem, therefore, that both low infant birth weight and birth defects might be associated with maternal weight before pregnancy.

At the moment these studies are based on animal research but human data may confirm this link, examining both the perinatal death rate and the infant abnormality rates in women whose body weights are well below those expected for their height, age and social class. Other obvious factors interact here too. Infection, smoking and alcohol consumption may be more common amongst women who have lower body weights. However it is probably that inadequate nutrition and low maternal weight before pregnancy is a major cause of low birth weight, miscarriage and congenital abnormalities. Maybe an improvement in nutrition to bring the underweight woman to a normal weight in this phase could help reduce problems in a subsequent pregnancy.

Special Cases

Some women may have different needs from the rest of the population. These can usually be identified well before pregnancy and help may be offered.

Vegans

A woman who is a vegan not only does not eat any meat but will not take any meat products either. Hence, she is excluding from her diet eggs, cheese and milk as well as meat. A vegetarian will probably take these animal products and will obtain all the essential primary amino acids, but a vegan will not take these contributions from living animals even when it does not involve killing them. Those who only eat food of plant origin often take in excessive quantities of cellulose, making them feel full very quickly. In consequence, they might not increase their calorie intake sufficiently. Further, some of the essential amino acids do not occur in plants; vitamin B12 and vitamin D intake may also therefore be inadequate.

Various tactics may be adopted. Vitamins can be replaced by man-made substitutes but it is hard to replace the essential amino acids. Comprehensive mixing of different protein sources may help but it is still difficult to get the primary amino acids. Mixing cereals with soy products and pulses is recommended to many vegan groups. In conjunction with extra portions of vitamin C-rich fruit (such as oranges) and folate-rich vegetables (such as spinach), this may help to reduce the deficiency. Sufficient calories may be gained by eating energy-dense foods containing vegetable oils and fats, such as chocolate, vegetable oils and salad dressings.

Food Allergies
Some people are allergic to certain foods. The immune defence system of the body is mobilized and if these foods are eaten unpleasant responses occur. Milk, eggs and wheat-based foods are the most common allergens. If the food intolerance is known about, it is wise for a woman to consult a dietitian in the prepregnancy period. Diets can be devised which are nutritious enough to cover pregnancy without involving the foods which stimulate the allergy. One of the hardest foods to avoid is milk and its products, for these are used in so many other foods. However, if an allergy exists, this can be done and extra attention should then be paid to providing alternative sources of calcium before the pregnancy period.

The Overweight Mother
Many women becoming pregnant are grossly overweight. Anyone who has a body weight more than 25% above the expected weight for a woman of her height may be considered to fall into this category (see Table below). Most women in this category can lose 1 kg (2.2 lb) every few weeks and so a woman who is 25% overweight should be persuaded to try and lose several kilograms before she becomes pregnant. This will give her a more comfortable pregnancy and delivery. Diets for this are the same as those for any other women who are overweight and copies will be found in many books on this subject. Indeed, there is much more written about weight loss in those who are overweight than about proper nutrition for those of normal weight. Advice should always be taken from the General Practitioner about dieting before starting a pregnancy.

Desirable Weights of Women According to Their Height and Body Frame (in Indoor Clothing Without Shoes)

Height cm (ft in)	Small Frame kg	(stones and lb)	Medium Frame kg	(stones and lb)	Large Frame kg	(stones and lb)
142 (4 8)	42–44	(6 9 – 6 13)	44–49	(6 13 – 7 10)	47–54	(7 6 – 8 7)
145 (4 9)	43–46	(6 11 – 7 3)	45–50	(7 1 – 7 12)	48–55	(7 8 – 8 9)
147 (4 9)	44–48	(6 13 – 7 8)	46–51	(7 3–8 1)	49–57	(7 10–9 0)
150 (4 11)	45–49	(7 1 – 7 10)	47–53	(7 6 – 8 5)	51–58	(8 0 – 9 2)
152 (5 0)	46–50	(7 3 – 7 12)	49–54	(7 10 – 8 7)	52–59	(8 3 – 9 4)
155 (5 1)	48–51	(7 8 – 8 1)	50–55	(7 12 – 8 9)	53–61	(8 5 – 9 8)
157 (5 2)	49–53	(7 10 – 8 5)	51–57	(8 1 – 9 0)	55–63	(8 9 – 9 12)
160 (5 3)	50–54	(7 12 – 8 7)	53–59	(8 5 – 9 4)	57–64	(9 0 – 10 1)
162 (5 4)	52–56	(8 3 – 8 11)	54–61	(8 7 – 9 8)	59–66	(9 4 – 10 5)
165 (5 5)	54–58	(8 7 – 9 2)	56–63	(8 11 – 9 12)	60–68	(9 6 – 10 10)
168 (5 6)	55–59	(8 9 – 9 4)	58–65	(9 2 – 10 3)	62–70	(9 10 – 11 0)
170 (5 7)	57–61	(9 0 – 9 8)	60–67	(9 6 – 10 7)	64–72	(10 1 – 11 4)
173 (5 8)	59–63	(9 4 – 9 12)	62–69	(9 10 – 10 12)	66–74	(10 5 – 11 9)
175 (5 9)	61–65	(9 8 – 10 3)	63–70	(9 12 – 11 0)	68–76	(10 10 – 11 13)
177 (5 10)	63–67	(9 12 – 10 7)	65–72	(10 3 – 11 4)	69–79	(10 12 – 12 6)

Based on information from *Human Nutrition and Dietetics* by Sir S. Davidson, R. Passmore, J.F. Brock and A.S. Truswell

Conclusions

Nutrition is concerned with eating but that is not all it is in the prepregnancy period. Nutrition is the planning of a sensible diet that will put you and your partner into the best state for the pregnancy that is to come. It involves some effort and planning but there are many good sources of information in public libraries. Probably the best technical book on this is *Nutrition in Pregnancy* by Bonnie Worthington-Roberts. This is a technical volume but it is well worth consulting because it contains much valuable information about the basic research on the subject. The best author of more popular books is Catherine Lewis who has written two paperbacks for the

National Childbirth Trust called *Growing Up With Good Food* and *Good Food Before Birth*. Both these books offer most useful and practical advice to the prepregnancy couple.

NINE

Tobacco and Other Addictive Drugs

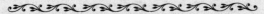

The inhalation of the noxious smoke of tobacco
weeds wastes and dries the body, consumes
the spirit and weakens the baby by corrupting
the very nourishment of the child in the womb.

After Culpeper*

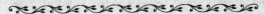

*AUTHOR'S NOTE: Tobacco smoking was almost unknown among women
when Culpeper wrote his book, so I have employed artistic licence, using his
words to express what I am sure he would have written.

Tobacco

Inhalation of the smoke from the smouldering dried leaves of the tobacco plant probably started amongst the American Indians in ceremonials when they were smoking pipes of peace. The plant and its seeds were brought back from America to Spain and thence to the rest of Europe at the end of the fifteenth century. Jean Nicot, who was the French Ambassador in Lisbon, sent tobacco seeds to Catherine de Medici, Queen of France, in 1560. From his name comes the word nicotine. Sir Walter Raleigh brought the leaves back to Britain and made smoking popular here. Whilst half the world's tobacco production is now in Asia, the largest single exporter is the USA which sells high quality Virginia tobacco, particularly to Europe. Other important tobacco exporters now are Turkey, Greece, Brazil and Indonesia.

All this amounts to an enormous industry and many young people have been led into the habit. In the early years smoking was mainly confined to men but over the last few decades an increasing number of women have taken it up. Since the Second World War intensive advertising has equated having a cigarette with relaxing from stressful problems, thus creating conditioned reflexes which are very difficult to break out of in one generation.

Why Smoking is Harmful

Tobacco smoke is harmful when taken into the body. Very little is absorbed through the surfaces of the mouth or nose;

most is assimilated when it is inhaled into the lungs. There are many hundreds of chemicals in the smoke, only a few of which can be considered here. Many of these constituents are probably harmful and one should not consider the only cause of problems to be nicotine or tar, although nicotine is the best known constituent. Nicotine is absorbed easily through the lungs by diffusion into the bloodstream; in the same way it can diffuse across the placenta to the unborn child. Nicotine constricts the blood vessels, particularly in the central nervous system. It may also affect the uterine blood vessels supplying the placental bed and so reduce the flow of blood there. Spasm of the vessels in the umbilical cord might cause reduced flow in the fetal circulation, leading to a lack of oxygen at the tissues.

The kick that some people get from cigarettes is often caused not by nicotine but by the burning products of tar. These aromatic hydrocarbons are formed from the incomplete combustion of the tobacco leaf and amounts vary greatly according to the type of leaf and how it is packed. All cigarettes in the United Kingdom are labelled with their tar content. These powerful aromatics could have an effect on the fetus by interfering with the transport mechanism of nutrients across the placenta.

Carbon monoxide makes up a large part of tobacco smoke, again because of incomplete combustion of the leaf. In some cases concentrations rise as high as 4%. Carbon monoxide gas is absorbed readily from the lungs and attaches itself to the haemoglobin molecules in the mother's blood, forming carboxyhaemoglobin. Concentration of the carboxyhaemoglobin may rise by 4% or 5% with each cigarette smoked. Carbon monoxide passes easily across the placenta so the fetal haemoglobin also becomes blocked and levels in the fetus can be 15% higher than those in the mother. By binding with the fetal haemoglobin in the red cells of the unborn child the gas is preventing oxygen being taken at the placenta, thus reducing the oxygen level of the fetus.

Any combination of these three mechanisms or others from the other chemical constituents might be responsible for the effects on the fetus. One thing is certain and that is that the effects are dose-related. The more cigarettes a woman smokes the more she is going to affect her unborn child. The fewer she smokes the less he will be affected, but only with no cigarettes will there be no effect at all.

What You Can Do

It is important that the risks of tobacco smoking are known to every woman and her partner. This is emphasized in a non-scary way at the prepregnancy clinic and one needs to understand the difference between the hazards for the woman's total life and those that exist for the unborn child. The best advice would be for the future mother and father to stop smoking completely. Short of this, any reduction is worthwhile.

The actual inhalation of cigarette smoke might be part of a wider psychological habit. Dependency often reflects other anxieties and cigarette smoking sometimes helps to improve relaxation and diminish mood changes which in their own right may be harmful to the future pregnancy. No woman should feel guilty about smoking, a habit that many others in modern society have acquired; but if she can give it up, so much the better.

In some cases there has been a previous problem in the pregnancy which some unthinking doctor has told the woman was 'due to her cigarette smoking'. However, there is little in reproductive medicine that can be said to be definitely due to one cause or another and the woman should never be black-mailed into feeling guilty about some event that might possibly have been caused by the smoking. The emphasis should be on the prevention of future problems rather than on harking back to the past.

Giving up smoking is very difficult. Often the woman and her partner will have tried in the past and failed. Yet it is interesting to note that more people succeed in giving up smoking in pregnancy than at other times. As many as 60% of women who try to stop smoking because of their future baby are successful, at least for the pregnancy and sometimes for ever. This success rate is three times greater than that among the non-pregnant for there is a much greater incentive.

All the problems of stopping smoking are well known and need not be reiterated here. Most women are helped at this stage by the fact that they are hoping to have a healthy child and that they are well motivated to look after that child in the uterus. Further, prepregnancy clinics are often couple clinics and so the partner can perhaps be persuaded to strengthen the woman's resolve by also giving up smoking. Encouragement from other members of the family and reinforcing the message by reading the relevant books and by visits to the clinic will all help. The exact technique used to stop smoking will differ from one woman to another and many organizations can help with this. Your local Citizens Advice Bureau should be able to help with addresses.

Case Study

Mrs U B was referred to the prepregnancy clinic from a Local Authority smoking clinic. She admitted to smoking forty cigarettes a day and wanted to break the habit for many reasons, one of which was that she was thinking of starting a family.

We explained the hazards which smoking posed to the unborn child and Mrs U B listened to them all. At the end she summed up by saying that if she went on smoking forty cigarettes a day it sounded as if she would have a smaller baby and that would probably be a good idea. We hastened to widen the discussion, hoping to change her views on this; we told her that it was not only the size of the baby that would be affected but also his development and capacity to grow up normally. She did not like this part of the advice but eventually absorbed it.

(Case Study cont.)

Mrs U B actually did give up smoking just before she became pregnant; she cut her consumption down from forty cigarettes a day to one after each major meal (three or four a day). She stayed at this level throughout pregnancy. It was difficult at first but she was able to use the pregnancy as the incentive to stop her smoking.

Eventually Mrs U B had a normal delivery of a 3 kg (6 lb 11 oz) boy at thirty-eight weeks. She was very happy and when we saw her at a gynaecological clinic for an incidental problem two years later she told us that she had still not started smoking again. Mrs U B attributed her non-smoking to the pregnancy and was glad she had stopped at that time.

The proportion of women in all age groups who are smoking has increased greatly; about 45% of all women in the United Kingdom had the habit in 1989. The problem is so great in the United Kingdom that lung cancer, an end result of smoking, will soon be more common amongst women than amongst men, who have always been the main sufferers of this condition in the past. Despite the long-known associations of smoking with serious diseases in the lungs, heart and blood vessels, it was not until the late 1950s that the effects of cigarette smoking on the unborn child were highlighted. Several studies in the USA and Britain in the 1950s and 1960s showed that a heavy cigarette smoker was likely to produce a small-for-dates and less mature baby. Some researchers also found an association with premature labour.

Smoking rates in pregnancy vary with the age and race of the woman. In the USA, where the background incidence of smoking in pregnancy was 26% in 1980, the lowest prevalence was in the Hispanic women; the black women had a rate of 26% and white women 29%. Similarly in the United Kingdom where the rate of smoking in pregnancy is about 37%, the prevalence is highest amongst the white women and lowest amongst the Indian and Pakistani population. In Islamic countries, smoking amongst pregnant women is almost non-existent; in developing countries it is lower than the Western world and in many European countries is less than 10%. However, tobacco consumption is increasing rapidly in developing countries and women are taking their share of this increase.

The age group which most commonly indulges in cigarette smoking is eighteen to twenty-four, the peak age of reproduction. There is also a trend to increased smoking with lower socio-economic class. In consequence, there seems to be a cluster of poorer, younger women who smoke more heavily than the rest of the population. About one-third of smoking women will stop during pregnancy and another quarter will reduce their consumption. Unfortunately, it is again the women over twenty-five years who are best at reducing cigarette smoking, whilst those in the peak reproductive group are more likely to continue their habits unchanged.

A large national survey organized by the National Birthday Trust in Britain in 1958 showed that if smoking was reduced or stopped before the sixteenth week of pregnancy (four months), then the outcome for the baby would be the same as for the non-smoking group. After this time, reduction in smoking has less effect. It might be argued therefore that the prepregnancy clinic is not the correct place to start propaganda about not smoking cigarettes, for the woman could stop when she knows she is pregnant and still have a good effect. However, breaking a habit like smoking is hard and takes time. It is best to clear the habit if possible before any pregnancy starts. Prepregnancy advice is intended to cover the whole pregnancy period and not just the very beginning. It is a time when a couple who want to learn about how their pregnancy may best progress want to hear about any relevant problems; it is therefore wise to include smoking advice at this stage.

Problems Associated with Smoking

There are many problems associated with smoking before and in very early pregnancy. The first is in achieving a pregnancy;

the second is in structural abnormalities of the baby which are laid down in very early pregnancy, often before the woman realizes that she is pregnant; then follow many other problems. In consequence, a reduction in smoking would benefit these two areas directly as well as having an effect later on in pregnancy.

FERTILITY

Smoking tobacco seems to impair a woman's capacity to produce a fertilizable egg and her partner's ability to produce sperm. For over twenty years maternal smoking habits have been correlated with infertility. An American study in 1968 showed that the percentage of infertile couples in the population was 14% among the non-smokers and 21% in the cigarette smoking group.

Cigarette smoking has also been associated with an increase in menstrual upset and with an earlier onset of the menopause when ovulation ceases. Researchers have calculated that women who smoke fifteen or more cigarettes a day shorten their potential reproductive life by 1.8 years compared with non-smokers. This might be due to a change in the pituitary hormone regulation of ovulation or a direct effect on the ovaries of the constituents of tobacco smoke.

About one-third of all infertile couples in whom a cause is found involve a male factor. Smoking men have a much higher percentage of abnormal sperm in their semen than do non-smokers. Since the journey of the sperm to the egg is very long it is only the most efficient sperm that get to the far end of the Fallopian tube. An increase of sperm abnormalities in the semen therefore reduces the effective sperm count. This is probably a direct effect of the nicotine itself on testicular tissue.

For these reasons it is suggested that both males and females are compromising their chances of getting pregnant by smoking. The best advice from a prepregnancy clinic would be to give up smoking before parenthood. The support of the other partner often helps at this crucial time and may lead to reducing or even stopping smoking permanently, a great advantage to all-round health.

CONGENITAL ABNORMALITIES

A survey in America in 1978 reported that the risk of abnormalities to the children of smokers is more than twice as high as that of non-smokers' children. This obviously also depends on other variables, such as the age of the mother, her past obstetrical history and socio-economic class. These studies have shown that if a woman who is smoking miscarries, the embryo, although chromosomally normal, is more likely to be congenitally malformed. It is therefore possible that in certain societies women who smoke are more likely to have malformed embryos. However, these are frequently lost in miscarriages and are therefore not counted in the statistics on babies at birth.

SPONTANEOUS ABORTION

Smokers are more likely to suffer miscarriage than non-smokers. This might be due to the increase in congenital abnormalities or the fact that smokers tend to include more women with other factors of differentiation such as poor nutrition or lower social class. Even when comparing women in equal jobs, with probably equally stressful environments, smokers still have a higher miscarriage rate and women who smoke also tend to go into labour earlier. If all else is normal this does not matter greatly and only curtails pregnancy by a week or so. However, if smoking is added to other detrimental factors, it may cause a very early preterm labour.

LOW-LYING PLACENTA

The placenta may be low sited or may be less well formed amongst smokers. One should be careful to remember that there are many factors that affect implantation, but smoking might have a direct effect through nicotine or its effect on the blood supply of the uterus. If tobacco smoke causes blood vessels to be slightly constricted, then the area where the ovum normally implants might be relatively less well supplied with blood. The lower part of the uterus (normally not as well supplied as the upper) may become a reasonable alternative site for implantation. As pregnancy advances the uterus grows, leaving a low-sited placenta and increasing the risk of placenta praevia*. Researchers have also described microscopic abnormalities of circulation on the fetal side of the placenta occurring more commonly in smokers.

PERINATAL DEATH

For all these reasons the perinatal mortality rate and percentage of low birth weight babies are both much higher amongst smoking women than non-smokers. Some scientists go so far as to say that 10% of all perinatal deaths of babies can be attributed to maternal smoking. Others consider this figure to be high but all note an association. It is also possible, however, that cigarette smoking is the outward sign of some difference in the woman's metabolism or personality and that is the real cause of the problem rather than the cigarette smoke itself.

LOW BIRTH WEIGHT

A smoking mother will have a smaller baby than a non-smoking mother. This is due in part to the lack of growth in the baby; the other reason is the almost double risk of delivering a baby preterm. A baby born to a woman smoking more than fifteen cigarettes a day will be more than 200 g (7 oz) lighter at birth.

Some women may consider this to be an advantage because delivering a smaller baby may seem easier. However, it must be remembered that along with the lower birth weight goes a lack of development. Such babies are more vulnerable to the hazards of low birth weight than a baby of equivalent weight from a non-smoking mother. Developmental tests performed at five, seven and eleven years after delivery show that the children of heavily smoking mothers come out much worse than those of non-smokers.

This might be an effect of the woman's personality and her social environment but smoking often stands alone as an independent variable in multivariant analyses. In the first year of life, babies of smoking mothers themselves have a 50% increased risk of being admitted to hospital with bronchitis or pneumonia. Neville Butler and Jean Goldstein reported their findings from 10,000 children in the 1958 National British Study and showed that, at eleven years of age, the children from smoking mothers still had deficits in reading comprehension and general ability, while their height was reduced compared with the children of non-smoking mothers.

Conclusions

It is difficult to prove cause and effect with smoking-induced problems, for the woman who gives up smoking is likely to be a more compliant person than the one who continues despite advice. Personalities, body build and body metabolism may all differ between the non-smoker, the smoker who is prepared to give up and the ardent smoker. Even if there was only a weak association, the prepregnancy counsellor should advise women of the short-term pregnancy effect and the longer childhood effects associated with smoking mothers. The aim is not to be a scare-monger but to inform mothers so that they are aware of the facts. If they still do not wish to give up smoking it would be wrong to dragoon them into doing so with horror stories. It has to be remembered that a woman who gives up smoking unwillingly may well develop further stress problems as she tries to stop smoking. These problems of stress might be worse than the effects of the cigarettes themselves.

Other Addictive Drugs

As our society becomes more aware and informed about drug addiction and the measures taken become less punitive, more women who are dependent upon drugs are coming forward for prepregnancy advice. Some of this guidance is given at the prepregnancy clinic but much of it is better given in drug addiction clinics in association with large hospitals. If someone seeks such advice at a hospital it would be wise to involve an obstetrician who could then sit in with the drug counsellor.

Opiates

The traditional addictive drugs, heroin and opium, have been less commonly used in the United Kingdom although they are now increasing and are rampant in other parts of the world. Law enforcement agencies and socially minded politicians try to get at the problem by reducing the sources of opiates and their transportation from one country to another. This still leaves the prepregnancy clinic with a few women who are addicted to heroin or, to a lesser extent, to other opiates.

Large studies, done mostly in the USA, have shown that such addicts have a higher risk of many obstetrical problems compared with control groups. For example, the perinatal mortality rate is two and a half times higher and preterm delivery rate is almost twice as high. There is also a five times greater risk of the baby being small for gestational age. All these differences may relate to the social and environmental background of the woman, her nutrition and her tobacco smoking habits as much as to the opiate.

Two other studies from the USA have shown there to be a threefold increase in the rate of multiple pregnancies among opiate users. This might be due to the ovary being stimulated so that extra follicles release eggs, or the hypothalamus might react with an increased gonadotrophin release.

Neonatal withdrawal symptoms occur within the first day of life in over half the babies born to heroin-dependent mothers. As the unborn child has become used to a certain level of heroin, when removed from that source by birth, he shows increased irritability, with tremors and sometimes fits. There is a problem with swallowing and digestion of food and occasionally there is respiratory distress so that the baby cannot breathe easily. Such babies have an increased risk of dying from Sudden Infant Death Syndrome (cot death). Again, there may be social factors which account for this increased risk but heroin and opiates do interfere with the mechanisms that control the heart and respiration. The baby exposed to heroin early in life may therefore have less stable control in the next few months.

In the prepregnancy period, the therapist should aim to

detoxify any woman who is on heroin and try and convert her to another less addictive drug, methadone. A methadone programme can be maintained and the woman is much less likely to have complications in pregnancy. Infants exposed to methadone in the uterus may have withdrawal symptoms that are more prolonged than with heroin but they are usually less severe.

Case Study

Miss P T was a registered heroin addict with a complex lifestyle. She lived in a squat and had been convicted several times for petty thieving to pay for her heroin. She slept around freely and did not admit to using contraception. She smoked cigarettes heavily and her diet was largely based on Mars bars. Considering that a pregnancy was probable, the medical social workers wondered if a visit to the prepregnancy clinic could do anything to help Miss P T, for in her good moods she was a very maternal young woman.

Miss P T took her heroin by mainline (intravenous injection) and was accustomed to two shots a day, with up to four on days when she could obtain extra supplies. She was reluctant to discuss matters with yet another doctor and so the interview proceeded rather as a monologue. However, she was agreeable to having a blood test done for HIV III*, a common complication of those who share the needles used for drug injection. We gave her an appointment for a return visit two weeks later, thinking we might not see her. However, Miss P T turned up, mostly out of curiosity for the result of the AIDS test, which was fortunately negative. She warmed to the nursing sister who managed the prepregnancy clinic and listened attentively while the sister pointed out the hazards to the unborn child of heroin. After two more visits Miss P T agreed to consider detoxification and went

(Case Study cont.)

with our prepregnancy clinic sister to a centre where she was weaned off heroin.

She became pregnant whilst on methadone, a much less severe drug than heroin with less effect on the fetus. There were some problems with intrauterine growth retardation in later pregnancy but these would have been much worse if she had been on heroin. She delivered a 2.3 kg (5 lb) boy at thirty-seven weeks. That child was eventually put out to foster and we have not seen Miss P T since.

This rather mixed case might not be considered a great prepregnancy clinic success but at least it showed Miss P T that she could give up for a time and allow the child to be born, uninfluenced by heroin.

Marijuana

Smoking marijuana (otherwise known as pot or hashish) is very common in the USA and fairly frequent amongst the young in the United Kingdom. Regular use of marijuana does not seem to have such severe effects as heroin but the pregnancy may be shorter and there is a decreased maternal weight gain. The newborn babies are often more irritable and easily startled as withdrawal of the marijuana occurs. As with other addictive drugs, one has to distinguish between the interrelated problems of marijuana intake, tobacco smoking and alcohol associated with malnutrition.

The marijuana user is difficult to detoxify. There are specific programmes run by many centres and she should be in touch with these. The prepregnancy clinic will advise where the nearest clinic is, but treatment involves many sessions and the motivation of such women is often not very great. If a strong bond forms between the counsellor and the woman this, in itself, can be an important factor in helping the woman to stop her marijuana intake. Of course there is also the desire to produce a healthy child but this may be less important to a woman at a high level of addiction.

Cocaine

Cocaine can be taken by injection or by sniffing. Generally those who use the former method are more addicted and harder to manage. The fetus seems to notice the cocaine very quickly, for pregnant addicts report increased fetal movements within a few minutes of taking the cocaine. The problem of apportioning the harm a particular drug does has already been emphasized; it is difficult to differentiate between the effects of cocaine and those of other addictive drugs taken concurrently such as alcohol and marijuana. Congenital malformations do seem to be more common, while the birth weights of babies are lower, but as has been stressed previously, this may be partly due to the social background of the woman who is using cocaine. If one matches women for age, numbers of children, socio-economic position, use of antenatal care, smoking and alcohol habits, the number of people left to study is very small. It would seem that cocaine-exposed infants have an eight times greater risk of weighing less than 2.5 kg (5lb 7oz) at birth. Their mothers have a higher incidence of premature membrane rupture, thus going into preterm labour more readily.

Any woman who is using cocaine intravenously (and the same applies to those using heroin intravenously) should be considered to be at high risk for AIDS. The sharing of needles is common in this group and blood to blood contact from somebody with AIDS is one of the most effective methods of transmission in the Western world. This is dealt with in Chapter 6.

Conclusions

The addictive drugs work by being taken into the bloodstream and then reacting and influencing the brain. Unfortunately they also go to all other organs and, in the case of the pregnant woman, to the unborn child by passing across the placenta.

Opiates can affect the baby in the uterus by causing growth

retardation, and it is likely that the child will suffer withdrawal symptoms after birth. Treatment for addiction can be given if the woman is seen in time before or during pregnancy, but many opiate addicts are unwilling to attend the clinic for care. Marijuana, commonly known as pot, has less effect in pregnancy, but may still reduce the length of gestation so the woman may produce a smaller baby, which may also suffer from withdrawal. Cocaine affects the fetus soon after the mother inhales or injects it. Congenital abnormality is more common in babies of cocaine-users and birth weights tend to be lower. In all cases, however, it is difficult to differentiate conclusively between the effects of the drug and the general effects of the woman's social background.

TEN

Alcohol Abuse

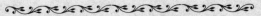

Let her drink moderately of clear wine, not
exercise too much, nor dance, nor ride in a
coach that shakes her.

Culpeper

Drinking used to be largely a male preserve but women in the Western world have now also taken to alcohol. In the USA alcohol abuse in pregnancy is considered to be the third leading cause of mental retardation after central nervous system abnormalities and Down's Syndrome.

Alcohol is a tissue poison. It interferes with the metabolism by depressing the action of all the enzymes in the body. Further, it is broken down in the liver into aldehydes* which are themselves metabolic poisons. Those who take alcohol in moderation may feel that it stimulates the body. It does this by removing inhibitions from the brain, thus releasing ideas and concepts which might previously have been repressed by the pressures of modern life. However, as anyone who consumes alcohol knows, after a few more drinks the consumer is past the stimulatory phase and into the depressive phase which gets worse with more drinking. At the cellular level there is no stimulatory phase; it is all downhill.

The prohibition of alcohol before and during pregnancy goes back to Biblical days. In Carthaginian law wine could not be consumed by a couple on their wedding night in case it caused defective children to be conceived. Aristotle considered that foolish, drunken women for the most part brought forth children like themselves, morose and languid. The Bible, always good for a reference on social habits, gives the following advice in Judges 13 to Samson's mother who is wanting to conceive: 'Thou art barren and bearest not, but thou shalt conceive and bear a son. Now therefore beware, I pray thee, and drink not wine or strong drink or eat not any unclean thing.' In Hogarthian England a committee on alcohol abuse in 1736 reported that: 'Unhappy mothers habituate themselves [to alcohol] and the children are born weak, sickly, often looking shrivelled and old as though they had numbered many years.'

Fetal Alcohol Syndrome

Over the years, mental defect and infants with 'a starved, shrivelled and imperfect look' have frequently been observed in alcoholic families. However, the subject has not been considered important in antenatal or prepregnancy care until the last two decades. Children born to heavy drinking mothers can now be recognized as suffering from Fetal Alcohol Syndrome. When babies are born they have growth retardation, central nervous system dysfunction and unusual facial characteristics, including very small eyes and a small head. A 1986 study from Britain reported that such a syndrome was found in 11% of infants whose mothers consumed two or three drinks a day through pregnancy. This incidence rose to 19% amongst mothers having four drinks a day and 30% for those who drank more than five drinks a day. All these groups of women who drink heavily would probably be included in less than 3% of the population of the United Kingdom at the moment.

Conversely, a study reported in Dundee in 1988 showed that there was no detectable effect on pregnancy from alcohol consumption below 100 g (3.5 oz) per week, equivalent to approximately ten standard drinks or one and a half drinks a day (see Box overleaf). In the Dundee study, 82% of women were taking less than one drink a day. By the time early pregnancy was established, 98% of women were below one drink a day and 45% did not drink at all. In later pregnancy, 65% of women reported they were not drinking and 32% were only taking one drink a week. Thus the vast majority had become virtually teetotal in late pregnancy but in early pregnancy there were still a small number (2%) drinking more than one drink per day, a group which before pregnancy had included 32% who had one drink a day or more.

Metabolism of Alcohol

Like cigarette smoking, alcohol is not an isolated feature of social life. Those who drink heavily probably also smoke cigarettes and may come from a poor socio-economic group, with a lower income and poorer nutrition. Large groups of women are needed if researchers are to assess each of the variables in order to examine alcohol in its own right.

Further, the reporting of alcohol consumption is not very precise. If a woman thinks her doctor is going to disapprove of something she may be economical with the truth about her real consumption. This is found when talking about food consumption to those who are overweight or the numbers of cigarettes smoked by those with a bad chest. Alcohol intake is therefore quite likely to be under-reported.

Blood tests can be used not only to estimate blood alcohol concentration but also to measure the breakdown products of alcohol. A woman consulting the doctor might not have had a drink in the hours before the appointment but the breakdown products reflect the drinking of twenty-four hours before and could thus be used to check the woman's own memory of her previous night's activities.

Alcohol is absorbed at many points in the alimentary tract, starting with the stomach and ending with the large bowel. As it is a small molecule it is absorbed fairly easily. However, if the intestine is working fast, or there is less blood going to the area at that time, absorption will be slower and peak levels will not occur so readily. Once pregnancy starts there is a delay in the emptying time of the stomach and intestines. A pregnant woman may therefore have lower peak alcohol values in the blood but the alcohol will remain in the body longer.

Checking your Alcohol Intake

When you drink alcohol it passes rapidly into your bloodstream and travels to the uterus. It crosses the placenta easily and thus enters the baby. Probably the best advice is to avoid all alcohol during pregnancy, for it is a tissue poison. However, for some women, who are used to drinking, this would be impossible and could increase the stress of pregnancy.

It is hard to measure your alcohol intake precisely but the following system is recommended:

One unit = one glass of wine
            or
            half a pint of beer
            or
            a single spirit measure

This rough rule will enable you to assess your intake. Out of pregnancy women should not drink more than fourteen units in a week and men twenty-eight units a week. This apparent chauvinism is due to the fact that women have a smaller body build and their tissues react differently to alcohol. Thus the non-pregnant woman could be consuming up to two units a day without putting herself in any great medical danger. However, in pregnancy it would be wise to limit this to one unit a day.

You must decide yourself on your level of alcohol intake, but even if you usually only take a little, do not have any great binges or consume enough alcohol to become inebriated. That excess might correspond with a crucial time in the development of the growing embryo and lead to an abnormality.

Other variables in assessing the effects of drinking in very early pregnancy are just as likely to confound the results. The tolerance of women to alcohol differs from that of men, for they have up to 30% fat in their tissues. This increased fat content in the female body absorbs alcohol and releases it later. In contrast, about 15% of male body weight consists of fat, so men can metabolize alcohol more readily. Once pregnancy has started, with the increased retention of water in the blood and other tissue spaces, a woman who is used to alcohol may have to take in much more to get the same social or psychological effect as when she was not pregnant. Alcohol is transported in water and is distributed through the body in proportion to the water content of various compartments. Hence, the unborn child will get a relatively higher level of alcohol, for his capacity to retain water is greater. Alcohol will be retained for longer inside the fetus than in the mother's circulation.

Some women have a habit of binge drinking. For example, they might absorb a very large quantity of alcohol on one occasion, such as a party or a lonely evening, but they do not have a large average daily intake. A very high blood alcohol level produced by binge drinking could affect the embryo at crucial points of limb or organ development (see Chapter 2). Further, the acidosis* in the fetal blood resulting from breakdown of the alcohol might affect the respiratory centres of the unborn child.

The breakdown of alcohol takes place in the fetal liver; in very early pregnancy there is no liver and even after it is formed at 4–7 weeks it is not very efficient at breaking down alcohol (for the maturation of enzyme systems there is very poor). Hence, the fetus would be at a double risk: concentrations of alcohol would be higher, whilst the breakdown rate of alcohol would be slower. Concentrations would therefore remain higher in the fetus for longer.

Case Study

Mrs G M enjoyed drinking alcohol in large amounts. She consumed over 60 units a week (the equivalent of eight whiskies a day) and often indulged in a binge at the weekend when she might consume a whole bottle of spirits in one evening. She was thirty-one years old and alcohol was not yet affecting her general health, although she did admit to feeling awful most mornings. She came to the prepregnancy clinic with a friend, who had attended for an entirely different reason. Whilst waiting outside Mrs G M saw a poster about drinking in pregnancy and then talked to the sister who told her about the clinic.

Mrs G M returned four weeks later to discuss her own position and the effect alcohol might have on her future family. We went into the details of her consumption and its probable effects on an unborn child. We also went into the problems of bringing up children afterwards and Mrs G M was shaken. She returned two weeks later and seemed willing to try to break herself of the habit.

We put her in touch with an alcohol counsellor in one of the voluntary organizations. She attended there reasonably regularly and after three months she was down to having one drink a day. Perhaps fortuitously, she then became pregnant and the surprise of that, in addition to the unwelcome words heard before, caused her to give up completely in pregnancy.

Mrs G M attended the antenatal clinic regularly and all went well until thirty-eight weeks when she had a vaginal bleed. A placenta praevia* was diagnosed, an event unrelated to her previous drinking. She had a Caesarean section under epidural* anaesthetic, producing a 2.8 kg (6 lb 4 oz) girl.

We last saw Mrs G M in the antenatal clinic in her second pregnancy two years after the events described. She told us she was virtually alcohol-free and was looking forward to a normal delivery of a healthy baby.

Why Alcohol Affects only some Mothers

It might be expected that if alcohol works as a chemical tissue poison, then the more the woman drinks, the more seriously her baby will be affected. This is not strictly so, for some women have babies who appear to be alcohol-affected even though they themselves are only mild drinkers, whilst other heavier drinkers seem to get away with it. The only absolute answer at the moment is that if someone drinks no alcohol, there is no effect.

Alcohol may have several effects on the unborn child. As well as the effect of alcohol *per se*, there is the possibility of damage caused by acetaldehyde, one of the breakdown products of alcohol made in the mother's liver. This product may pass to the fetus and perhaps cause fetal damage. Possibly those women who produce alcohol-damaged babies have got some fault in their own ability to break the acetaldehyde down into simpler products. In such women the fetus is therefore exposed to high concentrations of acetaldehyde. Further, those who drink heavily may have an inbuilt genetic problem. It may be that this genetic trait is accompanied by other traits which affect fetal growth and behaviour after birth.

As always, one must remember the enormous number of factors that can affect a fetus, of which alcohol is only one. A woman who is an alcoholic will undoubtedly have other behaviour patterns of eating and smoking which might affect the baby. In addition, she may come from a more deprived sociobiological background than other women, although this does not seem such a major factor.

Research in 1988 from Edinburgh University indicated that the chromosomes of the egg or the sperm might be affected by a high dose of alcohol at a critical time. Certain abnormalities are associated with the absence or malformation of a chromosome and this may lead to spontaneous abortion. The Edinburgh work showed that if animals were fed alcohol around the time of ovulation, there was an increase in detectable chromosomal problems. The dose used was a high one but mice metabolize alcohol much more quickly than humans. Therefore the Edinburgh group came out with advice that, during the week or so before ovulation in which a couple wish to conceive, the woman should avoid alcohol. This is strong advice based upon another species; there is no evidence of its relevance to humans.

How Alcohol Affects the Man

Excessive alcohol affects the man's capacity to reproduce in an obvious way – he is unable to perform intercourse. Erection cannot be maintained and so his inability to fertilize is immediately spotted. However, this is only a small part of the problem. If he is a chronic alcohol drinker he will have problems in maintaining an erection even when he is not under the influence. This will lead to chronic inability to penetrate and thus consummate intercourse.

A more subtle change may occur in some men. The alcohol or its breakdown product, acetaldehyde, may affect the production of sperm. Changes in the structure of sperm can be found in semen samples from people who drink heavily; there are fewer of them and they are not so active. Hence fewer can ascend the Fallopian tubes, and thus become available for fertilization, in those who drink heavily.

How Alcohol Affects the Child

There is an increased miscarriage rate among women consuming more than two drinks a day and this is still present even when adjusting for other variables such as the mother's age, how many children she has, her race, her smoking habits and previous miscarriages.

Babies from mothers who drink heavily are often born even shorter than their reduced weight would lead one to expect. Their eyes are rather small and set close together, and they are often irritable and poor at sucking on the breast. They may even have tremors and respond irritably to being picked up, with arching of the back and increased stiffness of the limbs.

Their birth weight is reduced in relation to their length of gestation and the same poor growth goes on after birth. In many children who are born small for dates, there is a catch-up growth if they are fed an adequate diet, but not amongst alcohol-damaged babies. Some would suggest that this implies cell damage inside the uterus; a smaller number of cells are capable of growing, even though nutrition is adequate after delivery. The head circumference is small and in animal experiments it has been shown that the relative number of cells in the brain is reduced.

As they get older there is poorer development in their comprehension, with a lower intelligence quotient which seems to persist into later childhood. Learning difficulties continue and the children have problems in concentrating. The head circumference stays small into later childhood and later life. They are more restless and generally sleep fewer hours than other children.

All these are reasons for couples to be careful about alcohol consumption before pregnancy starts since, in the early days, the woman might not be aware that she is pregnant. By the time she stopped drinking it might be too late and fetal damage may already have been caused.

What to do in the Prepregnancy Period

All this variable background is reflected in the conflicting guidance given in pregnancy about alcohol consumption; this leads naturally to the rather draconian advice given in the prepregnancy period: the only safe amount of alcohol that a woman before or in very early pregnancy can take is none. This is often unacceptable to someone who is used to having a glass of wine with their evening meal or after a day's work. It is much better to individualize; if a woman is used to drinking alcohol in small amounts and has not had any medical or psychiatric problems she will be advised that whilst no drinking is perfect advice, to take a little alcohol will probably do no harm during pregnancy. It is a question of how much she will be concerned by taking no alcohol; the anxiety which might manifest itself through chemical stress factors could end up harming the unborn baby more than the small amount of alcohol she might take.

Prepregnancy counsellors will ask any woman who comes for prepregnancy advice about alcohol consumption. It is such a common part of social life that people can easily forget. The woman can help by noting down in her diary what she actually did consume (honestly) in the week before her prepregnancy appointment. This will give a more precise answer. Be prepared to answer honestly about any episodes of excessive drinking at parties or when feeling depressed. Remember that this is a professional and confidential consultation between an enquirer and a medical adviser; the truth is essential for a full and adequate assessment of what is going on.

Conclusions

The ideal advice to a couple preparing for pregnancy would be to drink no alcohol. However, this might be hard in some circumstances so both the man and woman would be strongly advised to limit their intake. If they are drinking a lot it may be wise to use one of the special programmes available in many parts of the country to help people with drink problems. Alcoholics Anonymous (see Useful Addresses) run special groups for pregnant women and this may be of help to those who think they have a problem.

ELEVEN

Exercise and Stress

Now then, if the blood be cleansed of what offends it, or corrupts it before it be sent down ... to be conducted into seed, the children bred of this purified seed must needs be stronger and by consequence more subject to live. Moderate exercise of the parents conduceth much to the lives of the children.

Culpeper

Exercise

Exercise used to be something we did at school and gave up soon after. Most teenagers would play an occasional game of tennis or football, according to their taste, but that was all. By the time they reached the pregnancy age group, they were doing little formal exercise. In the last twenty years bodily fitness has become such an important part of many people's lives that it almost amounts to a revolution. At the upper end of the spectrum are the health clubs with their expensive jacuzzis and fruit bars, then come the aerobics classes run at workplaces, down to the solitary man or woman who starts the day with jogging or exercises. Many people in the pregnancy age group are now exercising strenuously by running marathons and playing competitive team games.

The effects of exercise *per se* in the period immediately before conception are not well known. Only a little research has been done on this, but many people ask questions about it in the prepregnancy clinic. So often when doctors do not know about something they play safe and recommend the minimum. Thus, only two specific sports are often recommended for those wanting to embark on pregnancy: these are swimming and walking. Neither of these are competitive, nor do they put any particular stress on the body; swimming is often considered to be a weightless exercise, for the weight of the body is borne by the water.

Other slightly more adventurous doctors let people continue with harder sports such as aerobics, tennis or running, provided the women are fit and used to these activities. The more physical sports with body contact are usually banned. These include skiing and horse-riding. Here the risk is not so much of continuing at speed, but of falling down or falling off. However, such falls might not harm a woman who is thinking of becoming pregnant. In some parts of East Germany athletic coaches actually encourage women to have a child in order to help them to realize their 'full sporting personality'. This is probably as specious a statement as that made by some music coaches who encouraged their charges to have sexual intercourse in order to develop their singing personality.

However, many examples do exist of people starting a perfectly normal pregnancy around the time of heavy athletic endurance. Although she did not know it, Ingrid Christiansen, the Norwegian marathon runner, was pregnant when she competed in the 1983 London marathon. Her baby boy was born months later and was perfectly normal. In the 1958 Melbourne Olympics, the Russian women's team won over twenty medals and it later transpired that many of them must have been pregnant at the time of their sporting victories. Little is known about the effects of exercise on miscarriage and pregnancy and much over-protective advice is given unthinkingly, but generally, if a woman is used to exercise, continuation does no harm. In this chapter we shall review what is known about the subject.

Effects of Exercise

FERTILITY
Heavy endurance sports undoubtedly affect ovulation. Like the dietary and body weight problems discussed in Chapter 8, intensive training, long-distance running and ballet dancing produce dysfunction of ovulation in up to 50% of women. This applies particularly if the women are under twenty-five years old and have had a late onset of menstruation. The balance of the pituitary gland with the ovaries is altered by the physiological changes of exercise, causing reduced ovulation. This

should only be a temporary matter, but the hormonal after-effects go on for much longer than the exercise. The imbalance seems to relate to the extent and duration of the exercise. If this is so, then moderate exercise need not be avoided by people wanting a pregnancy.

Case Study

Miss L R was a ballet dancer with a well-known London company. She was twenty-four years old and had started dancing as a girl of six. She now held an important place as secondary dancer in the company and was looking forward to rising higher. She had met a male dancer two years before and was contemplating marriage. She came to the prepregnancy clinic from the ballet company doctor, for she had not menstruated in the last eight months and was concerned as to how this might affect her future fertility.

We saw Miss L R and examined her carefully, performing a series of tests on the hormone levels. These confirmed that while Miss L R was capable of making eggs, she was suppressing this, for her weight was only 48 kg (7 st 7 lb), some 20% below that expected for her height. We discussed this with Miss L R and she accepted that her diet was a meagre one, just enough to provide her with the energy she needed for the hard exercise she was doing all day and in the evenings. However, she wished to keep her body shape in the conventional manner expected by her ballet master and so we left it there.

Three years later Miss L R came back to the prepregnancy clinic. She had fallen out with her ballet company and gone into private ballet teaching. Her lifestyle was more relaxed and she wished to reconsider our advice. By now, Miss L R was only 5% under her accepted body weight; she had started to menstruate the month before she saw us and all we did was guide her towards the right foods for a few months. Six months later she became pregnant and delivered a 4 kg (8 lb 13 oz) boy with the help of forceps. She now exercises, still more than most of us, but with a reasonable diet which maintains ovulation.

There is no evidence to suggest that exercise has any deleterious effect on male fertility; neither the sperm structure nor the performance of coitus seem to be affected and indeed some males would consider that they are the better for exercise. All the folk lore on this subject seems to point in the converse direction (i.e. to the deleterious effect of recent intercourse on sporting activities), but this is ill-researched and probably owes as much to fiction as it does to fact.

RAISED BODY HEAT

Exercise leads to raised body heat, particularly in the internal organs. In animals it has been shown that congenital malformations can follow excessive central core heats, but the temperatures have to be very high and they must occur at precise stages in fetal development. Heat affects the growing embryo or fetus more than the unborn child, for the embryo can only lose heat through the mother. If the mother's heat is set higher then the embryo will not be able to lose heat so effectively.

Vigorous exercise for long periods of time can raise central core temperatures. For example, if a woman exercised hard for 60 minutes she might raise her core temperature from 38 to 39°C. Occasionally, after extreme exercise such as running a marathon of 41.8 km (26 miles), the temperature can rise to 40°C. All these levels are well below the temperatures involved in experimental studies on other animals where malformations were produced. A more likely cause of high temperatures which might affect the fetus would be an illness involving high fevers, such as flu, in early pregnancy. Obviously it would be better to avoid such illnesses but in real life this is sometimes impossible.

In ordinary exercise, most women are very unlikely to raise the body heat to anything like the temperatures required to cause abnormality even if they were in early pregnancy and did not know this. The prepregnancy counsellor can advise women that this is not a major factor and exercise should not be stopped for that reason only.

OTHER PROBLEMS

Very early in pregnancy, the hormone progesterone is released as part of the ovarian response to fertilization. This damps down uterine contractions and helps to stop rejection of the early embryo. The ligaments that guard the joints are made of connective tissue which becomes slightly laxer and softer under the influence of progesterone. Hence injury may occur at a lower level of stretch than before pregnancy. Should a woman be doing extra exercise at a time of high progesterone levels, she is therefore slightly more vulnerable to problems with her joints and back. A woman should be warned of this at prepregnancy consultation so that she can plan for any events in the future.

Certain forms of exercise would probably be unwise in early pregnancy. Water-skiing is a popular sport, but when women water-skiers are being towed at 20 knots, the water passing between their legs may produce a vaginal douche effect. This can be countered by wearing tampons (as is done in international water-skiing teams) or a well-fitting tailored wet suit. It is probably wise to avoid water-skiing in the period before pregnancy.

Another minority sport that is best avoided in prepregnancy and early pregnancy is scuba-diving. Compression followed by too rapid decompression does produce gas bubbles in the blood, and these might also occur in the fetal blood. A small bubble could have a more serious effect in fetal than in adult circulation. Again, much more research is required in this area but until it has been performed, pregnant women would certainly be advised to avoid scuba-diving below 6 metres (about 18 feet).

Conclusions

Every woman has a different concept of heavy exercise. A prepregnancy counsellor should consider this in relation to the individual woman and the enjoyment she gets from this activity; enquiry should be made into her menstrual background and reproductive history. If menstrual irregularities are associated with exercise the woman would be wise to reduce exercise to a level when menstruation (and therefore probably ovulation) became regular again. The climate in which a woman lives would have an effect. In countries warmer than the United Kingdom the effects discussed would probably be more relevant.

The woman's past obstetric performance should be considered; she may have had spontaneous miscarriages or premature labours. The cervix may be incompetent, or she may have had a history of babies that do not grow well. All women in these groups should be cautioned more actively about the effects of exercise in prepregnancy and early pregnancy.

Generally, women can continue their exercise into the prepregnancy and pregnancy period. It would be helpful if they could exercise in order to get fit before pregnancy, provided the period of getting fit does not cause lack of ovulation. In pregnancy itself they can ease up a little and do less energetic exercise.

Stress

At the prepregnancy clinic the subject of stress is often brought up by couples as a possible cause of problems. They all know what they mean, but it is sometimes hard to differentiate stress from fatigue and hard work. It is important that if someone uses the word stress it means the same thing to everyone considering the problem.

Stress is one of these words left over from Victorian medicine when it was considered that all conditions could be treated at the level of their symptoms. Most of these words, such as miasma, or toxaemia, have now been replaced by more scientific accounts of the condition, but stress still remains. Perhaps this reflects how little we understand the physiology of stress. We all have our own ideas of what stress is but it is difficult to measure the effect of something so undefined on an event such as forthcoming pregnancy.

At work and in daily life we are subjected to psychological pressures. If we are able to cope with these pressures we feel we are working hard but are not in any way stretched. However, if we cannot cope with them, and they are building up on us, then the word stress enters the arena. A stressed person is someone who is being pressurized and finds that the resulting aggravation is beginning to affect their physical health. A common early symptom is that they wake up at about 4 a.m. thinking about the problem which is stressing them. With the problems of possible unemployment, and greater competition in the workplace, many women attend prepregnancy clinics wondering about the stress of their job and its effect on future pregnancy. It is very difficult to give precise advice here.

Case Study

Mrs O D was a qualified accountant. She was now head of a department in a busy London office where the frequent, rapid and accurate production of accounts was an essential part of the business. In consequence, since Mrs O D did not trust anybody as she might have, she was often still there at 10 p.m. checking calculations. She lived in a very pleasant country house in Essex, but even at 10 p.m. it was a one and a half hour journey, followed by another lengthy journey the following morning.

She and her husband had been trying for a pregnancy for eighteen months and had been investigated at the local infertility clinic. Nothing abnormal was found in either partner. She came to our prepregnancy clinic by mistake, for the appointment should have been made at our fertility clinic for a second opinion on fertility. However, since she was there, we had a discussion. We went through her lifestyle and asked the simple questions: 'Was she waking from sleep in the early morning?' and 'Was she carrying work home in her head at night?' The answer was affirmative to both these so we investigated her stress further. It transpired that she was under considerable pressure at work. Her job was getting on top of her and causing her to worry not just about financial affairs but also about her status in the firm; she was beginning to see threats from those colleagues she considered to be rivals.

We had two sessions with Mrs O D, the latter with her husband also. We explained the lack of precision in the field of stress and talked of the problems caused when jobs get on top of you. The couple went away and thought things over. They wrote to us a few months later, explaining that Mrs O D had given up her job in the City and was now running a private financial consultancy in Chelmsford. This was about fifteen minutes from her home; she was much more relaxed and the purpose of the letter was to tell us that she had just been found to be eight weeks pregnant.

One cannot claim an absolute cause and effect here, but it is an example of the way stress may affect reproductive function.

Some women may have specific emotional problems, perhaps related to a previous pregnancy when a baby may have died in labour or immediately afterwards. The mother's sense of guilt or anxiety about this causes stress in future pregnancies. Such problems of psychological stress are best dealt with by frank explanations of what happened. It is also helpful to discuss changes in management that can be used to bypass or guard against events which previously led to the specific problem. This can be done in particular cases and is a most effective treatment.

The measurement of stress has greatly occupied psychologists for some years, and they now have stress measurement methods which probably exceed their power to interpret the results. The 'Schedule of Recent Experiences' is a commonly used questionnaire employed to measure stress. Some of the questions are not very precise. For example, if a woman is asked about stopping work, there is no way of telling from the questionnaire whether the stoppage was a voluntary one, or was forced upon her by the family or was even due to being sacked. The reason might even have been a happy one, such as her partner getting a pay rise or the couple inheriting some money, thus enabling the woman to give up work if she so wished. All these are enormously important factors, but are not covered in such a questionnaire. Other questions use vague phrases such as 'change of health'. This can be interpreted in many ways by the person filling in the questionnaire, yet the observer scoring the item will give the same marks to a variety of different responses.

The other problem with such questionnaires is that they do not pay sufficient attention to the effects of more long-term problems. Lack of money in a household, being single, the number of other children in the house or inadequate housing – all can cause stresses not usually assessed in 'Schedules of Recent Experiences'.

It is very tempting to use stress as an all-purpose excuse for problems that women have in pregnancy. It has been loosely linked with infertility, early fetal loss and congenital abnormalities, but there are many complexities involved. Those research workers who have tried to sort out the tangled skein of the effects of stress admit that there is very little firm information. In consequence, it is hard to apportion the precise role that stress plays in the prepregnancy period.

Many in the psychological field divide stress into state anxiety, which is related to immediate situations and does not last very long; and fate anxiety, which represents a personality characteristic and means that the woman's anxiety will respond to many stimuli. This is akin to the difference between reacting to a tactical situation and to a strategic situation.

Freud said that anxiety started in the infant, following the stimulation which occurred at birth. Neo-Freudians, however, believe that anxiety originates in the social process, and that it can only start later in life when the young child realizes his helplessness or dependency. They claim that anxiety grows because of the threats and punishments issued to control the child's behaviour. Experimental psychologists consider that stress is an acquired emotion which reflects a tendency to try to avoid pain or painful situations. Hence, they argue that those who have been exposed to intense fears in early life are more likely to be predisposed towards stress, particularly in relation to obstetrics and childbirth.

Severe stress is associated with a stronger psychological anxiety, perhaps when women have a negative attitude towards their husbands or even their mothers. Such women may see themselves as dissimilar to their mothers; they are less likely to have planned their pregnancies, and are more likely to have a negative attitude if they do become pregnant. They tend to be more neurotic, more likely to have experienced unhappy homes in the past, and to have marital and economic problems in the present. They are usually less secure, less well educated, and more likely to have immediate relatives living in the locality.

Conclusions

In general, we all know what we mean by stress when we use the word ourselves, we know when we are stressed and we know how to avoid it. If it is not going to add too great a financial burden, the woman should take steps to modify her working hours or pattern of work (both inside and outside the home), even giving up paid work entirely if she wishes; stress might then be avoided in the prepregnancy period. However, breakdown in marriage, unemployment and bereavement are obvious examples of causes of stress which cannot be prevented or cured in the prepregnancy period.

The stresses related to work may possibly be circumvented by changing work habits or even workplace, but the prepregnancy counsellor has to be very careful not to advise people to take actions which they may regret if a pregnancy does not actually follow. It should be remembered that such advice could produce more stresses by removing the woman from a congenial atmosphere at the workplace where she enjoys having a regular social life associated with her work.

Most importantly, the prepregnancy consultation provides an opportunity for both partners to air their views on stress. A sympathetic obstetrician will encourage the couple to consider their respective stress factors and the very discussion may prove helpful and therapeutic. In addition, it may help to answer specific worries, thus removing a major source of problems.

TWELVE

Contraception

The instruments of generation are of two sorts,
male and female: their use is the procreation of
mankind; their operation is by action and passion, the agent is the seed, the patient blood;
so that the body of man being composed by
action and passion, he must needs during his
life be subject to them both.

Culpeper

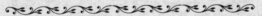

One of the most important aspects of bringing up a family is planning to have children at intervals that suit the whole family. Most couples are now able to have children when they want to, and not in a haphazard way. They can plan in a safe way by the sensible use of contraception. This should not be considered a negative aspect of life, but a positive one, which allows a couple to organize their children according to their economic and domestic commitments.

The United Nations, in its opening meeting in 1945, laid down four basic freedoms. They were: the freedom of speech, the freedom to worship, the freedom from want and the freedom from fear. Professor Sir Dougald Beard, one of Scotland's greatest obstetricians, considered that there should have been a fifth freedom and that was the freedom from unwanted childbirth. Since that meeting in 1945 many world organizations have tried to assist developing nations in setting up contraceptive programmes.

At the prepregnancy clinic couples often ask questions about the effects of contraception and the spacing of families on a future pregnancy. They are concerned that postponing having children might be a major problem; this is dealt with in Chapter 5. They are also worried about the effects of various contraceptive agents on future pregnancy.

Ideally, contraception should be a temporary mechanism, acting faultlessly with no side effects and reversible at the wish of the couple using it. In fact there is no such perfect agent – all involve some inconvenience or side effects. Most couples get their advice on contraception in the United Kingdom from a family planning clinic or from their General Practitioner. Different methods suit different couples, whilst the same method might not suit the same couple for the whole of their reproductive life. It is essential for a couple to stay in contact with their General Practitioner or family planning clinic to maintain continuity of advice as time goes by.

In the United Kingdom at present all professional advice and drugs obtained from the clinics or from the General Practitioner are free. Not all family doctors give advice but if your own does not, you would be well advised to go to another in the same practice who does. Some women may prefer the anonymity of the family planning clinic where they can see doctors and nurses specially trained in family planning methods, but who do not know the woman's background as well as the family doctor does.

Many couples attending the prepregnancy clinic are concerned with the effectiveness of contraceptive methods. How likely are they to prevent pregnancy? No method is 100% perfect and all have failure rates, either owing to the contraception being incorrectly used, or the body reacting to it in an unusual way.

The simplest measure of the efficiency of a given family planning method is the number of women who get pregnant per 100 couples using the method for a year. This figure is expressed as the number of pregnancies per 100 woman years. A good method of contraception would have a low rate, such as the combined oral contraceptive pill where the failure rate is 0.3 per 100 woman years. Less effective methods such as the non-careful use of the diaphragm or sheath could have a failure rate of 5 to 10 per 100 woman years. Unguarded intercourse produces between 70 and 80 pregnancies per 100 woman years.

Couples already using a method of contraception are often seen at the prepregnancy clinic. They are concerned about how easy it will be to stop this method, and what effect it may have on a subsequent pregnancy. There is far more folk lore than fact in many people's views on contraception.

Oral Contraception

Oral contraception may be a course of either combined oestro-gen-progesterone tablets or of progesterone alone. The former is known as the pill, the latter as the mini-pill. It is probably the most popular method of contraception used among young couples in the Western world; although it has been available for over thirty years it is still considered by many to be a relatively new method of contraception. When any complications do occur they are widely reported in the media.

Most oral contraceptives are a mixture of progesterone and oestrogen and are taken from the fifth to the twenty-fifth day of the menstrual cycle. When the pill is not being taken the withdrawal of oestrogen causes the lining of the womb to be shed and bleeding occurs. This method of contraception blocks production of certain hormones of the pituitary gland, in order to suppress the making of eggs. In addition, the pill may prevent the thinning out of cervical mucus at the time of ovulation, thus preventing most sperm from getting into the uterus.

The progesterone-only pills are useful if a woman cannot take oestrogen because, for instance, she is breastfeeding or is a smoker or is very overweight. They are not quite as effective as the combined pill, but they still give good contraception. A little breakthrough bleeding may occur; the mini-pill acts on the cervical mucus to prevent sperm penetration and on the Fallopian tube to prevent the assistance usually given to gamete* transport (see Chapter 2).

Anyone who is on the pill will have obtained it either from their family doctor or the family planning clinic. She should therefore return to them in the first instance to ask about the timing of oral contraception in relation to a subsequent preg-nancy. However some women do come to the prepregnancy clinic and whilst there raise points about oral contraception which need answering.

Generally speaking, if a woman stops taking oral contraceptive pills, their pharmacological effect ceases within two or three days. The liver can metabolize the hormones, oestrogen and progesterone, and if it is healthy, get rid of them as breakdown products. Seventy-two hours after stopping the oral contraceptive there should be no hormones left in the body.

However, the biological effects on the tissues may persist for as long as four to six weeks. It is therefore customary to advise women attending the prepregnancy clinic to stop the pill two or three months before they wish to conceive. This is not because of the hormones but because of the biological effects on ovulation. Having said that, many women become pregnant two weeks after stopping the pill, and produce normal babies.

Case Study

Mrs H J was a teacher with two children in their early teens; when she came to see us she was thirty-seven years old and had been on a combined oral contraceptive for six years. She came to the prepregnancy clinic because she was worried about what might happen if she got pregnant whilst she was still taking the pill. This had apparently happened to one of her colleagues at school and a termination of pregnancy had been recommended.

We discussed the matter with Mrs H J and checked which form of oral contraception she was taking. We went through the details of the timing of egg production and fertilization, and pointed out that if the combined oestrogen and progesterone pill have any effect it would be on the growing clump of cells in the first few days. This would either lead to complete rejection of the clump of cells, i.e. a spontaneous miscarriage, so early that she would not know, or it would have no effect on organ growth because no organs had been made at this stage. We also pointed out that many thousands of women had accidentally become pregnant whilst on the pill and had perfectly normal children.

(Case Study cont.)

After discussion Mrs H J felt happier about this and went away to continue her oral contraceptives for a few more years. We did warn her that after the age of forty it might be wise to consider dropping the oestrogen content of the pill and going on to progesterone only pills. We gave this advice because of the slight increased risk of thrombosis in people over forty on the oestrogen pill. She was glad of this guidance and said she would follow it.

The failure rate of the pill is very low, in the order of 0.1 to 0.5 per 100 woman years. The most common reason for failure is forgetting to take the pill. A small number of women get pregnant because the pituitary hormone still stimulates egg production despite the pill. Some of the women attending the prepregnancy clinics are afraid of what may happen if they get pregnant whilst on the pill. However, the doses of oestrogen and progesterone involved are so small that there is probably no effect at all on the developing embryo. There have been some reports of congenital abnormalities following the taking of the pill in pregnancy, but these are not substantiated. Recent studies have shown that there is no specific relationship between any type of malformation and oral contraceptive exposure.

Intrauterine Devices

It has been known for many centuries that a foreign body inside the uterus might affect the chances of implantation of a fertilized egg. This may be because of increased contractions of the uterus itself or a change in the consistency of the secretions, making it more difficult for sperm to travel up to the Fallopian tube or for the fertilized egg to come down and implant.

In recent years, the intrauterine device (IUD) became an important method of contraception but it is now slowly on the way out. The earlier devices were made solely of plastic and could stay in place for many years. Later ones had a coating of copper wire which increased their effectiveness and reduced their size. This was important for, whilst being as effective as the inert plastic ones, copper IUDs caused less irritation in the lining of the uterus, resulting in less heavy periods.

All IUDs are now under a shadow because of the frequency with which pre-existing infection or new infection flares up when these devices are used. In the next decade they will probably disappear because of the legal repercussions. The exception to this is when a woman has completed her family and merely wants to finish off her last decade of reproductive life. Then the IUD is a first-rate method because, having been put in place, it can be forgotten and the woman can continue her sexual activities without any concern that future pregnancies may result. Infection is also much less likely in this older age group (35–45) and if it does occur the results do not affect the woman's family potential.

Case Study

Mrs A F had read a lot about the damage caused by the Dalcon Shield, a form of IUD widely used in the USA and rather less in Britain. It had been withdrawn from use some years before because of its potential of allowing infection to ascend up the tail of the device from the vagina into the uterus. Mrs A F had a Dalcon Shield inserted in Canada in 1978 and it had been removed in Britain in 1982 because, in her case, it was associated with some extra heavy periods. She was now thirty-three years old and was concerned in case infection associated with Dalcon Shields might affect her.

We went into the matter in detail at the prepregnancy clinic and examined Mrs A F, finding no swelling or

(Case Study cont.)

tenderness in the region of the Fallopian tubes. We assured her that there was no evidence of any infection at the moment but she was very anxious to know whether the Fallopian tubes were open. We discussed the relative merits of doing a special X-ray (histosalpingogram) to check these and agreed that if she was still worried in six months' time, we would discuss this further with her.

Three months after the consultation she became pregnant and came to see us at the antenatal clinic. We were able to reassure her that this was the best test of patency of the Fallopian tubes, that a sperm and egg could meet and go on to produce an embryo. Mrs A F was happy with the result and went on to produce a normal boy at about thirty-nine weeks.

The IUDs generally have a low failure rate, about 0.5 per 100 woman years. Most failures are due to expulsion at the time of menstruation, usually very soon after the intrauterine device has been put in. However, a small number of women do get pregnant despite a properly retained IUD. This means that the physiological barriers set up by the irritating foreign body are not enough to stop the effective sperm passing through the uterus up into the Fallopian tube and causing a pregnancy. Likewise, these barriers have not prevented the fertilized egg from travelling down the tube and implanting.

Many couples are worried about a pregnancy starting with a foreign body in the uterus, especially as some early reports suggested that abnormalities could be produced by the copper-covered devices. However, more reassuring news has come from many larger, better-researched reports in which many perfectly normal children have been born to women who still have their IUDs.

If a woman does become pregnant with an IUD in place she is advised to contact the family planning clinic as soon as possible. Before twelve weeks of gestation, if the tail can be seen coming out of the cervix and if gentle drawing down on the tail allows the device to come out easily, it can be removed. After this stage of pregnancy it is probably wiser to leave the IUD in place. It does not have any effect on the growing baby and is often delivered after the baby in the placenta or the membranes.

The precise method of action of the IUD is not known. It probably works by irritating the lining of the uterus so that the fertilized egg cannot settle there. In addition, the smooth peristalsis helping the sperm up towards the egg is reduced by reflex action and interference with the muscle of the Fallopian tube. The copper-coated IUD may also have some chemical effect on the sperm while they are passing up through the uterine cavity. Usually a fine nylon tail is left trailing through the neck of the uterus into the vagina so that the woman can check for herself that the IUD is still in place.

Many women attending prepregnancy clinics are concerned that the IUD may have produced an infection that will prevent pregnancy. This might either be a flare-up of an already existing pelvic infection, or a new infection caused by bacteria ascending the tail of the coil. There is a small risk of this happening but it occurs mostly in the very young and those who may have had infections previously. The woman usually knows about it, for she has some pain in the side of the lower abdomen. Removal of the coil and treatment by antibiotics usually stops such infection and fertility is mostly unaffected.

When the woman wishes to become pregnant the IUD can be easily removed by gentle pulling down of the tail; an anaesthetic is not often required for this procedure. It would be wise to let a full menstrual cycle go by before trying to get pregnant in order to allow any uterine lining which has been irritated by the coil to be shed and replaced by a new lining in preparation for the fertilized egg.

Other Methods of Contraception

The diaphragm and the sheath used respectively by the woman and the man do not involve any prepregnancy problems *per se*. However, either may be used with spermicidal creams as are vaginal sponges, placed specifically for contraception. Couples attending the prepregnancy clinic have expressed an active interest in spermicides, for reports have associated such creams with an increased risk of spontaneous miscarriage and congenital abnormalities. In fact the number of babies in the reports was very small and the studies really showed the risk of poor reproductive outcome (rather than abnormalities) for women who used spermicides. Later studies showed no association between spermicidal creams and specific malformations but the fear had been raised in the public.

It is therefore wise for peace of mind to stop using vaginal spermicidal creams or sponges for one month before thinking of pregnancy, although there is no scientific proof that this makes any difference. This is a good example of a one-sided story being inflated by the media; when further and better evidence comes out this is not reported, for it is not considered to be news to the same extent as the bad news in the first report.

Many couples rely on methods giving knowledge of ovulation. The Billings Method, for example, depends upon the thinning of cervical mucus for a couple of days around the time of ovulation. Many women can detect this by self-examination. Taking the temperature every morning before getting out of bed can give some idea of the cyclical changes in a woman's basal temperature. The changes which occur around the time of ovulation may then be spotted on a temperature chart. Other couples use the Rhythm Method whereby they do not check mucus consistency or the woman's temperature, but just assume ovulation to be some twelve to sixteen days before the next period begins and so avoid intercourse around this time.

All these methods may have higher failure rates than the

pill or the IUD. However, when used carefully they are good contraceptive methods for a married couple having regular intercourse who pay attention to their own body functions. Such methods present no problems in prepregnancy.

Conclusions

The contraception problems that may arise in a prepregnancy clinic mostly fall into two groups. Firstly, there are the effects that a method of contraception used previously may have on a subsequent pregnancy weeks or months later. Generally speaking, there is little risk of such effects and the relevant details have been given here.

Secondly, there are problems relating to pregnancy occurring whilst that method of contraception is being used. Again, the information we have, mainly concerning oral contraception and uterine devices, is mostly reassuring. Perfectly normal babies have been born despite the correct use of these methods of contraception, so there is little cause for concern in this area. However, since it is wise to be certain, it is customary to leave the suggested intervals between stopping these methods of contraception and starting pregnancy in order to allow the body to return to its normal functions.

Section V

THE FORTHCOMING PREGNANCY
AND CHILDBIRTH

THIRTEEN

What You May Expect in Childbirth

When the child can no longer be contained in so small a place, the womb, by expelling faculty, sends it forth with great straining, and this is called travel or labour.

Culpeper

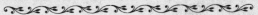

The Anglican *Book of Common Prayer* contains a special service for the thanksgiving of women after childbirth, called the Churching of Women. Many women's fears about labour are exemplified by a prayer which the woman recently delivered is advised to offer: '. . . humble thanks, for that Thou has vouchsafed to deliver this woman, Thy servant, from the great pain and peril of childbirth.'

Although nowadays many people do not attend church regularly, the thoughts expressed in this prayer still exist in the minds of many women. If such questions are concerning you, they should be discussed and fully aired in the prepregnancy period. You need not go through the anxieties of conceiving and pregnancy with false information about childbirth itself. On the whole, most childbirth these days does not involve 'great pain and peril'. The 'great pain' is dealt with by reasonable analgesia, offered properly by the staff looking after the woman. 'Peril' is something which has been reduced enormously in the last few years so that childbirth in the Western world is now an almost completely safe process. Unfortunately this is not yet the case in the developing countries.

Many women contemplating pregnancy are worried by stories they have heard about what may happen during childbirth. They may have heard tales, usually very embellished, of their friends' or relatives' experiences. Other women are worried because they themselves have had babies before and events did not go well. Such ideas can cause so much anxiety that the woman starts to dread pregnancy and refers to the prepregnancy clinic for advice.

If you have such concerns about a forthcoming pregnancy, a visit to your family doctor will often be enough to reassure you. Should the events of a previous pregnancy worry you, ask to see the obstetrician of the hospital at which you were delivered and he may be able to go through the case notes with you. It is essential not to bottle up these worries, thinking they will go away.

Obstetrical complications rarely occur in isolation; usually there are several problems to be dealt with and each ranks differently in priority. The whole situation would have been assessed by the doctor before a line of treatment was recommended and carried out. Hence, it could be misleading if you were to start seeking out answers to these questions by looking up medical tomes in the library or by asking your friends. All the combinations of variations in delivery are not covered in general texts which are intended to give an overall picture and then teach by considering the extreme examples. Further, your experiences are not the same as those of your friends and so you cannot automatically apply their experiences to yourself. Every woman is different and she therefore deserves a full explanation of the particular group of problems which led to the worry she is now experiencing.

The prepregnancy clinic provides an opportunity to discuss these matters; if you have an open access clinic near you, make use of it. This chapter gathers together many of the questions asked about childbirth itself (rather than pregnancy) at the prepregnancy clinics run by the author over the last few years.

Will my Baby be too Big?

Most women wonder how a 3.2 kg (7 lb) baby can come through the vagina, a tube with an internal diameter of about 2.5 cm (1 in). The vagina has a fibrous and a muscular wall; under the influence of the hormone progesterone, the muscle cells become extremely dilated so that by the end of the pregnancy period the tube is very lax and the fibrous tissue is very soft. In most women the vagina can stretch fairly easily to 10 or 13 cm (4 or 5 in) to allow the baby to pass down. Indeed, if this were not so, the human race would have died out many generations ago.

In addition to the elasticity of the passage, the baby passes down in the most efficient manner, packaging himself into the smallest possible bundle. The head is tucked well down so the chin is on the chest, usually leaving the smallest diameter of the baby's head – about 10 cm (4 in) – to present first. This causes no problem to most women with a normal vagina, the walls of which have been softened by progesterone during the months of pregnancy.

Some women are worried in case the baby is larger than usual. Whilst 3.3 kg (7 lb 4 oz) is the average for babies born in the United Kingdom, it is not unusual to have 3.6 kg (8 lb) or even 4 kg (9 lb) babies. These will deliver vaginally if the bony pelvis, made up of the mother's sacrum and the pelvic bones on either side, is of an adequate size. The soft tissues of the vagina are very rarely a deciding factor. If the baby's head will pass the bony canal of the pelvis, the woman, after a longer labour, can deliver even a 4 to 4.3 kg (9 to 9 lb 8 oz) baby. Once birth weight gets up to 4.5 kg (10 lb) the problem gets harder. If a woman has had babies before, she could probably deliver up to 5 or 5.4 kg (11 or 12 lb) but if it is her first baby it might be difficult and many women would prefer to have a Caesarean operative delivery to bypass this problem. A Caesarean section is readily available in all hospitals of reasonable size in which women deliver in the United Kingdom.

If the woman has had a very large baby before she will undoubtedly consider this in the prepregnancy clinic and wonder if the event will be repeated. In early pregnancy she must tell the obstetrician looking after her about the previous occasion and he will keep a special watch. He may need to get records from another hospital if the woman has changed addresses. If she is growing another large baby in this pregnancy, ultrasound tests can assess how big he is. If the doctor considers labour is going to be very difficult because of the large infant he will probably recommend a Caesarean section.

Usually a woman establishes a reproductive pattern and the birth weight of successive offspring are similar. However, each pregnancy is separate and the next baby might not be as big; the obstetrician therefore may decide to wait cautiously and see what happens in labour. If there is any delay in the head descending, a Caesarean section will be done in labour. This can be done very speedily in most reasonable-sized obstetrical departments.

When will my Baby be Born?

Some women, particularly those who have had babies prematurely before, are concerned about giving birth too soon. In the United Kingdom the majority of women give birth between thirty-eight and forty-two weeks after the first day of the last normal menstrual period. An ultrasound scan is done at most antenatal clinics to help localize the expected time of birth by measuring the size of the baby in the uterus. This is very helpful if there is any doubt about the regularity of menstruation or if the date of the last period is not known precisely.

It must be remembered that this expected date of delivery, even for those who are sure of their period dates, is only a sum of mathematical probabilities calculated from the dates of thousands of women who have had babies previously. It is like the bookmaker at the races who puts odds on the horses; the one most likely to win is the favourite but favourites do not win every race, nor do all women deliver a baby on their expected date of delivery. In fact 6% of women actually have the baby on that day but 90% have it within ten days before or after.

What if my Baby is very Small?

The major concern about the timing of delivery is when the baby comes too soon. An immature baby does less well in early life than does the baby who is quite mature. Many women are concerned because on a previous occasion they produced a very small baby. Perhaps the child was born very early, before thirty-two weeks. Or he might have been nearer term at thirty-six or thirty-seven weeks but the weight was very low, implying retarded growth inside the uterus following relative malnutrition of the growing fetus.

In the case of premature delivery there is an increased chance that the woman may go into labour prematurely again, for the condition can recur. It would therefore be wise to avoid as many activating influences as possible, for it is likely that such a woman's uterus is more sensitive and more easily stimulated. She should take careful advice from her prepregnancy clinic and plan to reduce her workload in the middle and later part of the next pregnancy. If the woman is working outside the home, this may need to be curtailed in some way; where housework is concerned, help may be obtained from family and friends. It would be unwise to plan any trips abroad, and long journeys inside the United Kingdom should not be contemplated in later pregnancy.

Any woman who has had a previous preterm labour should only consider booking for delivery in a hospital which can look after very small babies. She may be disappointed not to be able to go to her local smaller hospital but her baby has a much better chance in one that has good neonatal paediatric facilities. Around the time when she had her previous preterm delivery, it may be wise to rest even more and to avoid sexual intercourse which itself can be a stimulus to preterm labour at around this time.

In cases where the previous baby came more appropriately on time but was underweight for dates the woman may suffer from intrauterine malnutrition again. This is most commonly due to some reduction of the uterine blood supply to the placental bed from the uterine vessels. It cannot be overcome by taking extra food. Any woman so affected should consider the implications of this in the prepregnancy period. She should book for delivery in a hospital that can measure the problems of fetal growth during pregnancy; some large research institutes can now assess uterine blood flow in order to give her the best advice. The worst aspects of the condition may be circumvented but the couple must be prepared to go to a large scientific hospital for help. The mother should be prepared to go into hospital for a few weeks in later pregnancy.

If a woman who has booked at a local hospital does go into labour very early (say at thirty weeks), it may be necessary to transfer her before delivery to a hospital with better neonatal paediatric facilities. This is by far the best way of moving a small baby, for at that stage the mother is still the baby's own incubator. The child has the greatest chance if it is born in a unit with special facilities and can be cared for properly by neonatal paediatricians from the very beginning.

Similarly, the mother with rapidly rising blood pressure may be transferred for care not because the obstetricians and midwives at the local hospital cannot look after her, but to have the best environment available for the baby at his birth and in the hours after. The alternative, delivering the baby in a small hospital and then transferring the child by ambulance in a mechanical incubator, does not have such good results as transferring the mother and delivering her at the larger unit.

Will my Baby be all right in Labour?

Sometimes a woman has lost a baby in a previous labour and is worried that this might happen again. The prepregnancy clinic counsellors will discuss this with her to try and determine the reason for the problem. If it was one of major severity that might recur, a Caesarean section will probably be recommended on

262 · THE FORTHCOMING PREGNANCY AND CHILDBIRTH

the next occasion to bypass the risk of labour. If there was a non-recurrent problem, however, then labour could proceed and the mother and baby should be watched carefully.

The use of continuous heart rate monitoring is now widespread in Britain and this will probably be used for any woman who has had a previous problem involving the baby in labour. Some women are concerned that this is intrusive. Once connected to a fetal heart monitor, they feel anchored and the machine stops their capacity to move around. Some machines can be connected to a small wireless set no bigger than a personal stereo; the woman can carry this in her dressing gown pocket and move around the labour ward with her partner.

However, such telemetry equipment is not universally available and fetal monitoring may well mean that the woman will have to stay close to her room, in her bed or in an armchair close to it. She must weigh up the advantages of this method of guarding the baby's safety against the wish to walk around. Nearly always, when the balance is put that way, a woman realizes that the benefit to the baby is the more important.

Some women are concerned about the use of direct monitoring with an electrode pick-up from the baby's scalp. They are worried that the little wire electrodes may cause some harm to the baby's head. In fact the wire is finer than any needle used for injections, and the electrodes pick up a strong signal from the baby's heart to give useful information. The electrodes do not cause harm to the baby, as they are only in the surface skin and do not go any deeper into the head tissues.

Other couples express concern about the interpretation of the fetal heart rate traces, having been disillusioned on a previous occasion. Fetal heart rate trace assessment is not a precise science; like so much in medicine, it depends upon the person looking at the trace. Certain changes in the fetal heart rate are serious alarms, others are less serious. The action taken on a changing heart rate trace would depend on the doctors and midwives looking after the individual woman and on her particular circumstances. No rules can be laid down for all cases but the professional staff are trained to look after the woman and her unborn child *in toto* and the woman and her partner can therefore have faith in their actions. A couple could always ask the midwife or doctor what a certain change on a fetal heart rate trace means and they will usually get a good explanation which is tailored to the individual baby being looked after.

In some units, if the fetal heart rate trace is showing doubtful alterations, the state of the baby is rechecked by taking a small blood sample to check the oxygen level and acid balance of the blood. This is a much more precise scientific investigation and gives the attendants more information so they can advise the couple as to how labour is going. Again, this involves a very small pinprick, drawing a bead of blood from the baby. It is well worth doing when indicated by heart rate changes for the value of the information obtained from fetal blood sampling far outweighs any small moment of discomfort caused by the pinprick.

Some women are concerned about the impersonality of fetal heart rate monitoring. They tell their prepregnancy adviser that the last time they felt as if they were in a factory production line and the monitoring reinforced this feeling. One woman described it as being rather like broody hens in a line with machines attached to them so that 'when we were about to drop our eggs, the midwife came along and caught the egg, having left the rest of labour to be mechanically observed'. This, if true, would be an awful approach to labour and one that should not happen anywhere.

Most midwives and doctors when looking after labour use monitoring to assist their hands and eyes, not to replace them. It is a bad hospital unit that allows the machinery to take over. The few horror stories one does hear are well publicized, so the idea soon circulates that a certain hospital is high-tech and must therefore be inhumane. To have appropriate technology in a unit is wise; to use it to replace human skills is both unkind and scientifically unwise. There may have been some occasions like this or the stories would not have started; but there can be few obstetrical departments in the United Kingdom that really behave like this.

If a couple is concerned about the use of machinery the best advice is to request a visit to the unit they hope to go to for delivery. There they can talk to the midwives on the labour ward and actually look round. Most hospitals are quite open now and are delighted to show potential clients around their units (provided that time allows, as midwives may be attending other women who are actually in labour). The image put out by some detractors of the Health Services of high-tech battery-hen type systems is grossly false for the vast majority of hospitals.

What are the Risks of Losing a Baby?

Despite all the modern advances in obstetrics in the last twenty years babies still die occasionally. In Britain, the rate of loss of babies around the time of birth is about eight per 1,000 deliveries. In 1958 it was thirty-two per 1,000 deliveries so it has been reduced to a quarter in the last three decades.

Women who have previously lost a baby are naturally concerned about the next pregnancy. The first thing to do when a baby is lost is to get the details from the obstetrician concerned. At most hospitals now a consultant will see the couple within some hours of the baby's death and then arrange to see them again later when all the test results are available. Although it may be difficult to talk about these questions straight away this is the best time to sort out the problems, while the events are fresh in the minds of all the staff. Consultants are not robots and when a baby dies in a unit, all the professionals are deeply saddened. Doctors or midwives also feel grief, and the loss of a child has profound effects for some time on an obstetrical unit. However, further assessment immediately after the event has the very practical advantage that the notes and the results of investigations are all available within a reasonable time after delivery. A senior doctor can then go through and review the whole pregnancy and delivery with the couple.

If for some reason an assessment was not done in the

past, or if it was done and the couple have forgotten the details, they should seek further information before the next pregnancy. The prepregnancy doctor can either consult the notes if the couple come to the same hospital or write for reports and summaries to be sent from another hospital. This will, of course, provide secondhand information which is not quite as good as that given by those who actually looked after the mother in the pregnancy.

A review should take place and any possibility of recurrent events be discussed frankly. Certain conditions which may have arisen in the last pregnancy are non-recurrent and this can also be said very firmly. The odds of repeatable complications recurring can be openly discussed with the couple, so they know where they stand. The lines of management that might prevent recurrences or limit their effects can also be discussed. This may well mean planning ahead and making some changes in lifestyle during the next pregnancy. For instance, if the woman works outside the home this may have to be curtailed if she needs to be admitted to hospital for some weeks in later pregnancy.

Case Study

Mr and Mrs Q T came to the prepregnancy clinic in 1985 to enquire about what might happen in their next pregnancy. On the last occasion, in 1981, Mrs Q T had gone into preterm labour at twenty-nine weeks, producing a baby weighing 0.6 kg (1 lb 4 oz). The child had died on the second day from respiratory distress. Both Mr and Mrs Q T were still grieving for that child four years later and she was very frightened of what might happen on another occasion.

At the prepregnancy clinic we went into the situation fully with Mrs Q T and got her permission to write to the previous hospital. We obtained the notes and went through them in detail at the next visit. We found that in 1981 Mrs Q T had ruptured her membranes painlessly

(Case Study cont.)

and then gone on to labour. The baby had a difficult delivery and at first had not been expected to survive. Resuscitation was therefore not performed immediately and the baby was eventually transferred at the age of six hours to another hospital 32 km (20 miles) away for intensive care.

We were able to assure the couple that neonatal care had improved since 1981. We told Mrs Q T that she should deliver in one of the big district general hospitals which had a good neonatal unit. She would be looked after carefully and, if required, the paediatricians would be in the labour ward to look after the baby should he be born early. Further, care of the newborn had improved a lot in the intervening four years and steps would be taken to try to prevent respiratory distress. We recommended that if she wanted to start a family it should be soon, for the years were passing.

Slightly reluctantly, Mrs Q T followed our advice and appeared in the antenatal clinic four months later. We followed her pregnancy and at twenty-seven weeks admitted her to hospital, more for her own peace of mind than for any medical reason. After three and a half weeks, at thirty-one weeks, nothing had happened and she was happy to return home. In fact she continued to thirty-seven weeks when she ruptured her membranes painlessly and went into an easy labour. After four hours she produced a 2.8 kg (6 lb 4 oz) boy who has done very well.

The causes of death in the uterus around the time of delivery are many. About one-third of these deaths can be prevented and the risks of another third can be greatly reduced by employing alternative lines of management to bypass the risk time. There is, however, a core of deaths which cannot be prevented. This should be explained sympathetically but frankly to any couple so that they can decide for themselves whether they want to take the risk of this being repeated (with the mental trauma involved). Many couples are prepared to take reasonable odds and proceed with the pregnancy. They hope that the doctors and midwives will be able to manage events and so the risk is put to one side.

This area of prepregnancy care concerns few couples, for a very small number of babies die, but it is most important. Anyone who has been involved with the loss of a baby will know the assurance they can get by attending and discussing a previous stillbirth or neonatal death with professionals.

How Will I Cope with the Pain of Labour?

One of the most common ideas in childbirth folk lore is that labour is painful. This has been passed on from generation to generation down the ages. Anyone who deals with animals will know that birth is occasionally accompanied by discomfort but when things go normally they very rarely seem to experience the pain which humans have during childbirth. Some attribute this to the conditioning of the human mind to expect pain, others to the changes in the bony pelvis that have come over many thousands of years from standing upright rather than leaning forward as other primates do. Be that as it may, it must be accepted that uterine contractions in labour are painful to most women. However, in the modern obstetrical hospital, the pain can be greatly reduced, as millions of women will attest.

Case Study

Mrs J W was referred to the prepregnancy clinic by her General Practitioner. She had had a delivery two years before after an extremely painful labour and this experience still frightened her. We went through the details with her at the prepregnancy clinic and asked for a copy of the notes from the other hospital. When these arrived we saw Mrs J W again and went through them with her.

According to the other hospital records, Mrs J W had been offered pain relief but had refused it on three separate occasions during labour. When we asked Mrs J W about this tactfully her jaw dropped and she suddenly remembered that this was actually true. It all came out then that she had talked with a neighbour about a week before the labour and had been told grim stories about the effect of the pain-relieving drug pethidine on the newborn baby. This conversation had impressed her so much that in labour she refused all pain relief, not just pethidine. When the baby was born she had a complete memory block about this and it was not until we asked her specific questions that she remembered it.

We reassured Mrs J W that many people do have such blocks and this was nothing abnormal; she had just put it completely out of her mind. She felt a little shamefaced about this but we tried our best to reassure her. We then took her up to the labour ward and showed her the various methods we use now. We were able to let her talk to women who were having epidural* analgesia during strong labours and she realized how comfortable they were compared with what she had been through.

She asked if she could come to our hospital when she did become pregnant and have the same pain relief. We were able to arrange this and when Mrs J W came in labour a year later she had an epidural which gave relief within twenty minutes. This covered the rest of the seven-hour labour with two top-up injections and she delivered herself safely of a 3.5 kg (7 lb 12 oz) girl. She was very happy with the epidural and has since recommended it to all her friends. We knew this because four other people in her road have turned up at the antenatal clinic, all asking for epidural labour pain relief.

The pain of childbirth is different from that of toothache or a broken bone, for in childbirth something wonderful comes as a result of the pain. Giving birth to your baby who will be with you for the rest of your life is something which many women consider more than compensates for any pain during the hours before delivery. It is remarkable how, in the days following, many women will deny the severity of the pain which independent observers would have judged to have been enough to be remembered certainly for many months. Childbirth is different from any other process and the compensations of having a baby are in themselves excellent pain relief.

In addition, obstetricians and midwives now realize that the woman who understands what is going on and knows something about the processes of labour is likely to be more at ease and even a little more relaxed. She will proceed through labour in an easier way than a woman who is ignorant of what is happening and is frightened about the unknown. Antenatal education is very important for understanding the events of labour. In the Western world hospitals run classes designed to help the woman and her partner get the hang of what childbirth is about, and there are numerous books on the subject. None of this can of course replace the actual practical experience of having a baby. Uterine contractions can be painful but it is possible to overcome this pain and the end result is well worth it.

At the prepregnancy clinic women often ask whether pain relief is needed in labour. Pain is an individually felt sensation, and what is painful to one woman may not be as painful to another. In addition, other thoughts in the brain can sometimes reduce the way the pain is perceived. Some women wonder if they can go through the whole process using relaxation methods alone. However, by the time labour is well advanced, most women wish for pharmacological pain relief. This can come from injections, nerve blocks or inhalation. Injections of pain-relieving substances like pethidine act by suppressing pain perception in the brain, while nerve blocks such as epidurals anaesthetize the nerves as they leave the spine, thus blocking the sensation of pain. Both of these are available in larger hospitals. In addition, a woman may breathe in a mixture of nitrous oxide and oxygen to get short-term relief from pain. The last method is not normally used until the pushing stage of labour, for it cannot be used for long.

Pethidine

Pethidine is a strong pain-relieving medicine. It is usually given by intramuscular injection in the buttock or thigh and makes labour much more bearable without making the woman unconscious. There is a slight relaxing action also, so that the neck of the womb opens a little more readily. Usually two or three injections will be required in the course of a first labour, but fewer in subsequent deliveries.

It is wise not to give pethidine too close to the baby's birth if this can be anticipated. The drug passes across the placenta and if the baby is born with a lot of pethidine there could be some suppression of early respiration due to depression of the respiratory centre of his brain. This does not affect the baby in the uterus, for then he is living on oxygen supplied from the mother across the placenta. However, after delivery the brisk action of the respiratory centre is important, for the child has to breathe on his own.

Pethidine is usually given by the midwife only when she is sure that the cervix is opening and the woman is really in labour. A few women do feel a little nausea and so an anti-nausea substance is often given at the same time as the pethidine. Many women who have benefited from pethidine in labour swear by it, for it produces a slightly detached but conscious mother in whom pain is greatly reduced.

Epidural Anaesthetics

The use of epidural* anaesthesia has expanded in the United Kingdom in the last thirty years. A local anaesthetic is injected through the back into the base of the spine so that the nerve roots are blocked where they leave the spinal sac. (This is not a spinal anaesthetic, an entirely different procedure, in which some local anaesthetic agent is put into the fluid which bathes the spinal cord.) An epidural is a much safer anaesthetic and produces pain relief swiftly for three to four hours. Because labour usually lasts longer than this it is often necessary to top up the dose of anaesthetic; in consequence most anaesthetists will run a fine plastic tube into the epidural space outside the spinal cord so that the next injection can be given into this tube, thus saving the mother another injection.

An epidural anaesthetic has to be administered by a skilled anaesthetist. Unfortunately, such doctors are not available everywhere, and so most epidurals are given in obstetrical units in larger hospitals. If the woman particularly wants an epidural, she should talk to her doctor and midwives. In a 1984 survey, just under 1 in 5 women in the United Kingdom used an epidural to cover labour. In some larger hospitals the anaesthetic can be guaranteed because there are enough anaesthetists on duty, day and night, whenever you arrive in labour. In others this might not be so, and there the obstetrician would be wrong to promise a method he could not supply. If you were keen on an epidural, it might mean changing your booking to a larger hospital and this may have to be arranged by your obstetrician if it is possible.

The disadvantage of an epidural is that, as well as blocking pain in the uterus, it also removes sensations so the woman cannot tell when the contractions are coming; pushing in the second stage of labour may therefore be more of a problem. This nerve block can be overcome by a good midwife or doctor who sits with the woman with their hand on her stomach. When the uterus contracts the professional observer acts as the sensor for the woman. They let the woman know when the contraction is there so that the pushing can sometimes be as effective as without the epidural.

However, this system is not as good as that which the body provides and in consequence there is a higher rate of forceps deliveries in association with epidural anaesthesia. This is not a serious thing in itself because forceps or a vacuum extractor can help the baby out, as is explained later in this chapter. With an epidural anaesthetic already running in the system this is not felt by the woman and so is not painful, but an operative delivery may frustrate her own wishes about how she was going to deliver.

Nitrous Oxide and Oxygen

The inhalation of nitrous oxide and oxygen is a good method of pain relief. It works very quickly, for absorption of nitrous oxide in the lungs is almost immediate and the analgesic swiftly reaches the brain. The effect occurs within seconds and some women cannot take more than a certain amount of nitrous oxide. In consequence, the self-administering inhalers are arranged so that the face mask has to be held in place; if the woman becomes too dizzy, the mask will automatically come away from the face. Nitrous oxide and oxygen mixes are very good analgesics in the second stage of labour and many women have benefited from it.

Some couples at the prepregnancy clinic are concerned that nitrous oxide may be harmful to the baby. It would be if it were breathed in as a pure gas, but it is used in the United Kingdom as a 50% mix with oxygen, thus allowing over twice the concentration of oxygen normally breathed from air. Since the analgesic is a gas, it is expelled via the lungs and this allows very rapid clearance if concentrations rise. (This is an advantage not found in analgesics administered by injection.)

The baby is usually well supplied with oxygen if the mother is breathing nitrous oxide and oxygen. It must be stressed that it would be unwise to attempt to use nitrous oxide and oxygen for the whole of a labour which is several hours long. This would cause an imbalance of the respiratory gases which could lead to serious side effects. Such overbreathing would blow off the carbon dioxide. While this does not matter for a few minutes, it would be harmful over a few hours, for it could cause a serious change in the acid–base balance of the blood.

Other Methods of Pain Relief

Much interest is now expressed in prepregnancy clinics about non-pharmacological methods of pain relief and how they may affect the unborn child. If one has faith in any method it will undoubtedly provide some pain relief, partly by the psychological overlaying of ideas and possibly by the release of natural body analgesics or endorphins from the brain. The non-drug methods have variable responses. Few women find such methods as psychoprophylaxis enough for the whole of labour but the techniques often work in early labour, thus postponing the time when the first formal drug analgesic has to be given. In consequence, at the prepregnancy clinic most women are advised to look at these other methods and investigate whether they suit them. There are many places where couples can learn about these techniques; the National Childbirth Trust (see Useful Addresses) has very effective tutors in these aspects of analgesia.

Psychoprophylaxis aims to reduce tension in the body by relaxation, controlled breathing patterns and concentrating the mind on something other than uterine contractions. Hypnosis works if the woman is susceptible to the process and if the hypnotist is prepared to stay with her for the whole of labour. Transcutaneous nerve stimulation with small doses of electricity is also a helpful method. It has been tried in many centres and provides help for some women in the early stage of labour. For others pain relief may last further into labour. It probably works by distracting the woman's mind from the pain of contractions but may also be due to the electrical nerve stimulation causing the release of endorphins, natural analgesics made by the body.

All these methods have advantages but all should be discussed beforehand with the midwives and doctors who will look after you in labour. It is far better to talk about what you are going to do with the staff looking after you. On the whole, the professional staff will be sympathetic to these methods and interested in helping you try them. Occasionally you may meet an obstetrician who suggests that you should not use such non-drug methods. If this happens you can try to move your booking to another hospital although this might be difficult; if the obstetrician is being adamant it is often not just because he is being bloody-minded. Possibly he has seen the method fail in the past and does not want you to be disappointed. However, if you want to persuade him that you would like to try it, and will not be disappointed if it does not work, he may well offer you the opportunity to use it.

If you do not want to use any drugs in labour, you can do exactly as you wish. Nobody is going to force you to have pain relief but it is probably wise to keep an open mind and be prepared to accept drugs if the pain of labour is more than you expect. Should you need help, it is not an admission of failure; no matter what degree of training or preparation for childbirth you have had, analgesic drugs may still be required for stronger contractions.

If you do ask for pain relief in labour, remember it will take some time from the request to the actual time of pain relief. If pethidine is required, the midwife has to be given the key to get the drug from an especially secure cupboard which is used in all hospitals for storage. The injection must be drawn up and checked by two qualified people (midwife or doctor). It is then injected into the muscle and takes about twenty minutes from then on for enough pethidine to be absorbed into the blood to have some effect on the brain. Similarly, an epidural request means locating the anaesthetist, getting him to the labour ward and then the insertion of the plastic tube. Through this the injection is made and pain relief comes some eight to twelve minutes after that. In either case, from the request to effective pain relief will take some thirty to forty minutes. You are therefore advised not to wait until the very last minute before requesting analgesic help. Ask for it when you first think you may want it.

Occasionally there has been disagreement between partners in previous labours and it is wise to try to ensure in the prepregnancy time that you and your partner are of one mind about this. There is nothing more distressing to the professionals than seeing passionate debates between the partners as to whether or not the woman should have pain relief. The professional can advise the woman generally but it is she who is going to receive the treatment. For many women labour is probably one of the most satisfying and exhilarating experiences that can be helped by modern, scientific pain relief, and no one should deny herself, or be denied, the methods of pain relief available if she requires them. By the same token, no women should be forced into taking any drugs if she and her partner definitely do not want them.

What Happens in Operative Deliveries?

Most women deliver normally with the baby coming head first, his chin tucked well against his chest and the smallest diameter of his head presenting to the vagina. He proceeds down the vagina propelled by the mother's efforts and uterine contractions. Delivery is normal and all are happy. In a quarter of deliveries in the United Kingdom, however, assistance is required. If she had had an operative delivery before, the woman often comes to the prepregnancy clinic asking about the chances of this being needed next time. Occasionally there have also been problems during the course of delivery and the woman must know the risks of a repetition would be reduced by a different method of delivery next time. More rarely problems have arisen in the long term after operative deliveries and, again, the couple at the prepregnancy clinic is concerned about these.

Forceps Deliveries
The most common method of operative assistance is with obstetrical forceps. These instruments have been used for over 300 years and have saved many babies' lives. The instruments

have been very skilfully designed and modified over the years. They may appear large but the head parts of the forceps blades are very slim – 2 or 3 mm (or ¼ in) only – and just slip in easily alongside the baby's head with a limited closing action. They cannot crush the baby's head but actually protect it by preventing the vaginal tissues from pressing on the head too much. Forceps look long but most of the blades are not inside the woman at all – only the part that is round the baby's head. The rest of the forceps remain outside the body, allowing the doctor to work with the mother to help the baby deliver.

Once the cervix is fully dilated the baby's head usually advances with contractions and maternal pushing. If it does not do this after a series of contractions, progress may have stopped, often due to an incomplete flexion of the baby's head. This would be all right for a short time but, if allowed to go on, it could lead to the death of the baby and eventual rupture of the mother's uterus, through continually pushing against an obstruction.

In consequence, the doctor may decide that the baby should be delivered. Further, in the second stage of labour the baby may be showing signs of distress with oxygen levels falling and the heart rate changing rapidly. All this will be explained to the mother but it means the baby should be delivered rather more swiftly than her natural efforts would allow. The doctor therefore guides the pair of carefully constructed metal shields or blades on either side of the baby's head, enabling him to deliver the child. It sounds like a forcible procedure but, with modern anaesthesia, most women experience no more pain with forceps than they do with a normal delivery.

Vacuum Deliveries
Another way of helping the baby out is by using a vacuum cap, made like a beret and about 5 cm (2 in) in diameter. This is placed on the baby's scalp and a negative pressure is applied inside it to raise the skin of the scalp into the cap. This allows a grip to be obtained on the head so that the

doctor can gently guide the baby's head down.

The vacuum extractor is used for a baby showing signs of trouble either at the end of the first stage of labour when the neck of the cervix is not quite fully dilated, or after full cervical dilation in the second stage. In the first instance it would be dangerous to use forceps, and vacuum extraction is much swifter than doing a Caesarean section. The vacuum (or ventouse) is a very useful instrument in the hands of those who are experienced in its use; indeed, in some parts of mainland Europe it has completely replaced the forceps. The baby born by vacuum may have a red ring on the skin of the head where the cap has been. This causes no harm and fades within a few days. If people are worried about this at the prepregnancy clinic it is usually explained that it is better to have this small red ring on the outside of the scalp than damage inside the skull, affecting the baby's brain.

Case Study

Mrs R J was very worried because three years before one of her neighbours had a baby born 'by a vacuum cleaner' and that child had 'an enormous bruise all over its head'. She wanted to know whether this method of delivery was still used and if so, why, when it caused so much damage.

We went through the points Mrs R J raised and it was obvious she was talking about vacuum extraction. Here, a small cup is put over the baby's head, usually on the back. A negative pressure raises the skin of the scalp into the cup, allowing the head to be guided down. It is used in 1 to 2% of deliveries in the United Kingdom. We discussed the technique with her and pointed out that a very small number of babies did have some bruising afterwards but it always healed; this bruising was outside the skull and not of the brain.

Mrs R J was still dubious so we took her to the ward and introduced her to a mother who had been

(Case Study cont.)

delivered by vacuum extraction two days before. Mrs R J was most surprised that the baby had nothing more than a pale red ring where the cap had been on the head. She was reassured that if her next baby should need a vacuum extraction, he would be no worse off than the baby she had just seen.

Caesarean Section

When a delivery cannot proceed vaginally, even with assistance, then a Caesarean section must be performed. If a baby has to be delivered in a hurry in the first stage of labour, before the neck of the womb has been fully dilated, it usually means a Caesarean section. This is an operative procedure performed by a skilled obstetrician under anaesthesia. They may use a general anaesthetic so that the woman is asleep, or an epidural anaesthetic which completely numbs the lower part of the body. The most common reason for doing a Caesarean section is when the baby shows signs of lack of oxygen during the first stage of labour. Less usually, the obstetrician may find that the baby's head is not fitting well into the pelvis so that progress is slowing or has even stopped; it would then be dangerous to continue attempting a vaginal delivery.

Women who have previously had a Caesarean section are often concerned about having another operative delivery. There is an obvious risk of this if the condition which led to the first Caesarean section is still in existence. For example, some change in the mother's pelvic shape may not have allowed the baby's head to fit well into the pelvis. This usually recurs from one pregnancy to another and it would be wise for the woman to deliver all her children by Caesarean section unless it was known that they were very small. However, many indications for Caesarean section, such as a lack of oxygen in the first stage of labour, are not recurrent and such a woman can often try for vaginal delivery the next time. Speaking generally, about one-third of women who have had a Caesarean section on a previous occasion deliver vaginally on the next delivery in the United Kingdom. Elsewhere, as in the USA, professionals hold the opinion that once a woman has had a Caesarean section she must always be delivered that way in subsequent pregnancies. In the United Kingdom this is considered over-dogmatic and over-protective.

After Caesarean section, there are sometimes post-operative complications; women also ask at the prepregnancy clinic about the causes of these and the likelihood of their recurrence. Any incision on the abdomen will be slightly painful but the pain is not usually enormous and it gets better in a few days. It is important to remember that people who have operations are generally unwell beforehand and are rather older than those having babies. Those who have a Caesarean section are usually fit, young women who have got nothing wrong with them and so their incisions heal quicker and better. There may be some mild problem with passing urine or opening the bowels for a few days but it is usually coped with by the woman with the help of the midwife. The presence of a healthy, active baby in the cot alongside the bed is the most useful aid to healing.

Caesarean section is a clean operation and the incision on the abdominal wall nearly always heals very well. Many surgeons now perform a curved smile-shaped incision at the lower part of the abdominal wall where the pubic hair will regrow. In consequence, the scar cannot be seen after a few months. A small number of women may have some infection of the wound or bleeding afterwards and this would lead to a less clean healing. There may even be some parting of the wound edges and this could result in a rather uglier scar. If this is in the lower pubic hair area it still would not show but can be unpleasant during the healing period. Generally, however, Caesarean scars are very secret and even repeat scars are well hidden, for the surgeon excises the previous one.

Very rarely, women undergoing Caesarean sections notice some pain during the operation itself. This has received a lot of publicity in the newspapers in the past but is very uncommon.

In a Caesarean section, the anaesthetist has to be certain that not too many drugs are given before the birth of the baby, for these could depress the baby's respiration when he is born. In consequence, a slightly lighter general anaesthetic than is employed in general surgery is used for Caesarean section until the baby is born. This is deepened immediately afterwards to allow the surgeon to proceed with the closure of the uterus and the wound. A few women may remember hazy impressions of what is said and done in the early stages of Caesarean section before the actual incision. Often this is not painful but rather like a bad dream. If some chance word or thought triggers the memory after delivery, the response of pain is maybe recalled. Like all dreams it is hard to be precise and most women do not remember the images, which follow the lighter anaesthesia given to guard the baby.

One way to avoid this would be to use an epidural anaesthetic for Caesarean section, for this provides the same level of pain relief throughout. This method is best used for non-emergencies (i.e. elective Caesarean sections), for it is not easy to put an epidural in swiftly enough for an emergency Caesarean section. For the planned Caesarean section, however, an epidural is a very good method of pain relief since it has little effect on the baby's capacity to breathe.

Another advantage is that the mother is awake and can take part in the process of delivery. In most hospitals, her partner can come in and sit at the top end of the operating table, talking to her while the operation proceeds. An epidural anaesthetic allows much more participation in delivery; the woman can hold the baby within seconds of birth, and is often breastfeeding the child while the abdomen is being sewn up. This may sound rather strange but such operations are happy family events at which the surgeon feels privileged to be present. An epidural takes some of the sting out of an elective Caesarean section.

Case Study

Mrs C W came to us at the prepregnancy clinic because she had had a Caesarean section eighteen months before to deliver a 3 kg (6 lb 11 oz) girl, following a lack of advance in the first stage of labour. She had an epidural anaesthetic and described the operation as being excellent. She felt no pain but was fully conscious when her baby arrived and was able to cuddle the child within a minute or two of birth, even while the surgeon was still proceeding with his work. Mrs C W was worried for she had been told that she would need a Caesarean section if she became pregnant again. Having read newspaper reports of a particular case, she was concerned that she might get a general anaesthetic which would allow her to feel pain but not to protest about it.

We discussed the matter in full and pointed out that since she had had a good anaesthetic on the previous occasion, she could ask for an epidural next time. She had not considered this point and was relieved by it. We had to tell her, however, that epidural anaesthetics were not universally available in the United Kingdom and she would have to book into a hospital that provided twenty-four-hour service. This would mean one of the larger units where they had enough anaesthetists and Mrs C W asked if she could possibly come to St George's Hospital. Since she lived 113 km (70 miles) away, on the other side of the River Thames, I suggested this was not a wise plan but that there were plenty of other good, large hospitals nearer her home. Together we looked up the names and addresses of some of them and she went away to plan her next delivery feeling much happier.

Will I Bleed at Delivery?

Every delivery is accompanied by a slight loss of blood when the separation of the placenta from its bed allows a few millilitres of blood to escape. Additionally, a woman may have a tear split at the entrance of the vagina or she may require an episiotomy (a releasing cut) in the same region. From this a few more ml of blood also escape. In all, most women will probably lose 150–200 ml (5–7 fl oz) of blood in a normal delivery. This is minute compared with the volume of blood which has been building up during the pregnancy and most women would not even notice this amount of blood loss. Occasionally, however, there is a greater loss of blood. Doctors and midwives are on constant guard against such a problem in labour.

Heavier blood losses may occur because the uterus is not contracting down on the placental bed. Blood therefore continues to flow from the placental bed immediately after delivery or from some split in the uterus, the cervix or the vagina. In a very small number of cases, heavy blood losses after delivery may be due to faulty clotting mechanisms preventing the blood from coagulating properly. These only occur in a very small proportion of women and they usually know about the condition beforehand. Such heavy blood loss cannot usually be predicted. For this reason many obstetricians and midwives are fearful, for the woman's sake, of deliveries conducted outside the hospital; there they cannot cope efficiently with such blood loss.

Because of the risk of postpartum bleeding occurring unexpectedly, all women delivering in the Western world are now offered an injection immediately the baby is born. This injection, an oxytocic drug*, helps the muscles of the uterus to clamp down firmly on the blood vessels going through to the placental bed. This is the primary method of stopping blood loss and the most important way of preventing haemorrhage. This injection has been used since the 1950s in the United Kingdom and is now customary in the management of normal women. Of late, there has been some debate about its effectiveness and necessity but at the moment there is no evidence that it causes harm and plenty that it does good. Certainly, any woman who has had more than usual loss of blood after delivery on a previous occasion ought to accept this injection for without it she could lose much blood and become ill.

Some women are at higher risk for postpartum haemorrhage and often come to the prepregnancy clinic to discuss the problem, particularly if they have had a previous delivery accompanied by a haemorrhage. The largest groups are the women who bled in a previous pregnancy because the uterus did not contract down on the placental bed or because of faulty clotting. Whatever the precise cause, the fact that there was a previous haemorrhage indicates that they should deliver in hospital where the medical and midwifery staff will be an extra guard against a heavy bleed happening a second time. Such women may have some laxness of the uterus – either inherent looseness or because they have had many deliveries and the uterine muscle is not in such good tone as it once was. The neck of the womb may have torn or the uterus may not have retained the separated placenta for long enough to contract down properly on the blood vessels going to the empty placental bed. All these are major causes of postpartum haemorrhage and can be guarded against in another pregnancy.

If there has been a large blood loss on a previous occasion, the prepregnancy counsellor will go through the events, sometimes writing to the hospital concerned to obtain notes in order to explain events more fully. In the next pregnancy the obstetricians and midwives will be even more on the alert to prevent loss of blood occurring. They will watch the uterine contractions carefully and will provide an injection which helps the uterus to contract down and stay contracted. They will watch very carefully for splits of the tissues in the genital canal and will deal with them swiftly as they happen. Also, in case blood loss becomes heavier, blood will be grouped and cross-matched so that it is available for the woman if necessary.

Case Study

Mrs B T had had her last baby at home two years before. She had a planned home delivery; all went well in labour and she delivered a healthy son. However, immediately after delivery she had a large blood loss. The hospital team had to be called out and Mrs B T was transferred to hospital by an emergency ambulance with a blood transfusion running. Although she did well afterwards she was severely shocked by the whole occurrence. Mrs B T was, to use her own words, 'terrified that this might happen again'.

We discussed the last delivery with her and went into the details. We pointed out that on another occasion she would have an intravenous injection after the birth of her child to cause the uterus to clamp down, thus preventing blood loss before it happened. We strongly advised her to deliver in a hospital which had good facilities.

Mrs B T fully understood the first point but was a little reluctant about the second, for she wanted another home delivery. However, on balance, she accepted that she ought to be under good care, having had a previous postpartum haemorrhage. She went away a little happier knowing that there was something that could be done.

Mrs B T booked with us and delivered about eighteen months after the prepregnancy clinic visit. She had intravenous syntometrine given at the time of delivery and her blood loss was minute. She and the baby went home twenty-four hours later.

There is a slight increase in the risk of haemorrhage occurring after delivery if the woman has had such a bleed before; for this reason the prepregnancy counsellor will urge the woman to take sensible precautions in the next pregnancy. She should enter labour in the best possible state and this is ensured by the doctors checking that she is not anaemic on arrival in labour. Eating the correct foods and maybe taking extra iron tablets in pregnancy will ensure this. During labour itself, special precautions will be taken.

If the blood loss exceeds 600 ml (1 pint) or so, the woman may need a blood transfusion from the stores in the blood bank. Of late, people attending prepregnancy clinics have been concerned that this blood might be a vehicle for AIDS. This fear is unnecessary in the United Kingdom where all blood donated for transfusion is tested for AIDS. There is no evidence in the last few years of women receiving blood in the United Kingdom which carried AIDS. Unfortunately, such reassurance cannot be given about all blood transfusion units outside the United Kingdom, and the woman should make her own enquiries about blood in other countries.

Some women have said they would like to have their own blood or that of their partner (if he is of the correct group) stored before delivery. However, this is not very practical; nobody knows the exact time of delivery and the blood may well be out of date before the baby is born, for its shelf life is only five weeks. Further, only 600 ml (1 pint) of blood can be taken from any given donor. If the woman bleeds heavily she would therefore require much more blood than this from the transfusion unit. It is best to rely upon the safety of the system rather than trying to make *ad hoc* arrangements.

Sometimes a woman has lost a volume of blood or clots some weeks after delivery and is concerned about this on a future occasion. This is usually due to a mild infection in the uterus and should be reported to the obstetricians during the pregnancy. Arrangements will be made then to check for an infection immediately after delivery and to offer appropriate antibiotic treatment if it is required. This too has a slight risk of recurrence and should therefore be discussed fully in the prepregnancy period.

What if the Baby Does Not Breathe?

After birth, most babies take in a big breath and then exhale, crying as they do, within thirty seconds of delivery; by one minute 96% of them are breathing spontaneously. The process of starting to breathe is one of the most complex physiological acts that the human body has to perform. The baby has been on the passive receiving end of oxygen and nutrients coming across the placenta for many months. Suddenly the lungs, which have had nothing to do during pregnancy, have to provide all the oxygen. In the last few weeks of intrauterine life they start to limber up and periods of fetal chest movements can be measured in the uterus. These preliminary rhythmical expansions are going to develop into regular respiration after birth.

At birth the child is subject to numerous stimuli. The cooling effect of coming from inside the woman's body to the outside world occurs despite the best of warm wrappings. Light and sound appear, the former for the first time and the latter much more intensely than inside the uterus. The effect of gravity is felt for the first time (in the previous months the fetus has lived surrounded by fluid in his private swimming pool and has been in a virtually gravity-free environment). In addition, the shut-off of oxygen from the placental supply means that the oxygen concentrations in the blood go down sharply; this is rapidly detected by the chemoreceptors in the baby's heart and blood vessels. The oxygen reduction is accompanied by an accumulation of carbon dioxide which causes a change in the acid balance of the blood; this too is detected by the physiological receptors in the baby's own circulation. All these activate very swiftly and most newborn babies cry and start to open their lungs within seconds of birth. A very small number will require help.

If a child does not breathe soon after delivery he is going to suffer from oxygen deprivation; the doctors and midwives in attendance will try and prevent this. The sucking out of the mucus and amniotic fluid from the back of the throat and nose is in itself a stimulus helping the baby take the first breath. If this does not work, then the attendant may have to pass a small tube through the back of the throat into the larynx, bypassing the vocal cords. This is connected to an elasticated bag which can provide oxygen at low pressure. On this intubation system, a baby can be kept well oxygenated by the professional for a long time before further help is obtained.

All this requires skilled obstetricians, paediatricians, midwives and equipment close at hand. It is one of the emergencies of obstetrics and professionals are trained to cope with it. A baby properly oxygenated by intubation usually does well; one that cannot be intubated does not.

If a woman has previously had a baby with respiratory difficulties she must be sure that she books for delivery in a centre where there is good neonatal care. A paediatrician will then be on hand for her delivery and all the obstetrical and midwifery staff will be aware of the past problem so that they can prevent or correct it if it happens again. This is an essential aspect of preventive medicine which can be planned carefully if the prepregnancy clinic's advice is taken.

Conclusions

Most deliveries are very happy events and almost all the problems that can arise may be prevented or overcome by modern obstetrical teams. If a woman is worried about any aspect before pregnancy, she should ask for professional prepregnancy advice. This is particularly true if there has been a previous delivery in which a complication occurred.

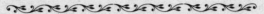

Good women, I have traced the manner we were made of to what we were when we were but an embryo. I have instructed you in its nourishment and growth in the womb. I have given you help for the preservation of it there.

Culpeper

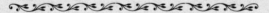

Conclusions

This book covers the areas in which prepregnancy care can be useful as well as those where prepregnancy care cannot be of help. At times existing research data has been misinterpreted by enthusiasts, and it is hoped that *Preparing for Pregnancy* has helped to clarify such issues.

The first few chapters gave an account of early embryo development, considering the problems which can arise. Chapters 4 and 5 dealt with problems we can do little about but must accept. The genetic background of a baby is dictated by the father and mother almost equally. Their individual lives up to this time are things of the past and cannot be changed, but the chances of these previous life events affecting the future child were examined.

Chapters 6 to 11 discussed the various aspects of contemporary life which could be modified if we want to help the development of a future child. A small number of women in the pregnancy age group may have had a chronic illness. These illnesses, and the drugs used to treat them, were discussed in Chapter 6. The effects of variations in normal life were then examined, including the problems associated with work. The influences of diet, smoking and alcohol were also detailed, and the less precise areas of exercise and stress were touched upon.

The common anxieties associated with contraception or previous pregnancies were considered in Chapters 12 and 13. Advice about the next pregnancy inevitably has to be of a general nature; couples are advised to talk to their local obstetricians for more detailed guidance on specific management.

Using proper prepregnancy advice, a couple should be able to plan their reproductive future with more precision than they could previously. In some areas, risks can be mathematically defined and indications of these given to couples. However, it is usually necessary to attend special prepregnancy clinics in order to get such information.

Much general prepregnancy education could be passed on through properly orientated teaching in schools. Later on, a couple will have to seek around for information and ask specific questions of their family doctors. If the results are not precise enough they can go to the special prepregnancy clinics that are now held in most regions of Great Britain. Here they will get a more precise answer to their question if a mathematical answer is known. They must realize, however, that we still do not have the answers in some cases, for medicine is an imprecise science.

The prepregnancy counsellor will probably not be able to tell them in detail what management might be expected in the next pregnancy. To find this out, they may want to talk to the obstetrician at the hospital where they are going to book for care in the next pregnancy and confinement. He or she will have views on the management of certain conditions, modified according to the population looked after and taking into account the facilities available. For example, the couple might want to ask what would happen if the woman enters a second pregnancy and develops raised blood pressure, having had severe hypertension in the first pregnancy. In such a case much of the general information about hypertension can be obtained in a prepregnancy clinic and most women are satisfied with the general discussion of the risks and possible managements. However, specific managements vary greatly and can only be described by the obstetrician who will actually look after that woman. Early contact would help.

It is hoped that what you have read here will help you progress through pregnancy in a happier and more relaxed frame of mind. The ultimate answer to all pregnancy problems is a healthy baby taken home soon after delivery. *Preparing for*

Pregnancy has been written with this aim, to let you know what the odds are on problems that seem to loom large in your mind now but may be really small to the baby when it arrives.

Glossary

ACIDOSIS The body fluids which bathe the tissue cells are virtually neutral in their acid-alkaline reaction. However if oxygen shortage occurs, the bias moves towards the acid side producing acidosis in body tissues and the blood.

ALDEHYDES When alcohol in the body is metabolized by being broken down, some of these breakdown products are aldehydes. They are toxic to body tissues.

AMINO ACIDS The basic building blocks of protein are the amino acids, fairly small molecules that can be constructed in various ways to produce different proteins.

AMNIOCENTESIS In order to obtain fluid from around the growing fetus, a fine bore needle is introduced through the mother's abdominal wall and the uterus into the amniotic sac. Amniocentesis involves the removal of a small amount of fluid for the examination either of the fetal cells for chromosome abnormalities or for the biochemical changes in the fluid associated with some fetal diseases.

AMNIOTIC FLUID The unborn child is surrounded in the uterine sac by amniotic fluid which buffers the child from physical jostling and temperature changes. The fluid is produced partly by the baby and partly by the mother.

ANAEMIA The oxygen-carrying function of the blood is performed by the red blood cells which contain haemoglobin. If they are deficient then we become anaemic. Their level can be detected very easily by simple blood tests.

ANTENATAL CARE A system whereby well women are screened during pregnancy by doctors and midwives in order to detect problems with the mother or the unborn child before or as soon as they arise.

ANTIBODY Whenever foreign proteins enter the body they are sopped up by antibodies produced by the immune system. If our immune response is not working properly then not enough antibodies are made and so the foreign protein can overpower the workings of the body. After a foreign protein has been in contact with the body, the antibodies it causes last for a variable amount of time, sometimes for life, e.g. the Rhesus antibodies among immunized Rhesus negative women.

ARTIFICIAL INSEMINATION The commonest form of artificial insemination is when the sperm is introduced into the upper vagina or cervical canal by a doctor using a syringe. The sperm may come from the husband (AIH) or from a donor (AD).

BASES The processes of respiration, muscle action and food metabolism in the body can lead to the production of certain acidic compounds. These are neutralized rapidly in the body by bases, such as bicarbonate and some of the protein molecules in the blood.

CELL The cell is the individual building block of the body. All organisms are made up of a series of various kinds of cells linked together to provide a working organism.

CHORIONIC VILLUS BIOPSY To detect changes in the chromosomes of the unborn embryo, a little tissue may be removed at about ten weeks of pregnancy from the edge of the placenta before it is finally formed. This tissue contains the chorionic villi which are minute fragments derived from fetal tissue. They may be examined for chromosomal abnormalities.

CHROMOSOME The genetic pattern which is passed from parents to child is stored in the nucleus of every cell of the body. There it is in the form of coded chemicals lying along long spiral ladder-like structures grouped into chromosomes. There are twenty-two pairs of chromosomes in each human nucleus plus extra ones for each sex.

CILIA In many parts of the body a current of fluid through a tube is whipped up by large numbers of muscular hairs protruding from the cells lining the tube. These all beat in unison and cause the material in that tube to pass on. Cilial action is essential in many parts of the body, such as the air tubes to the lungs where the current moves sputum in one direction, and in the Fallopian tube where they help pass the fertilized egg down towards the uterus.

CLOMIPHENE Occasionally the ovaries need stimulating to produce eggs. One way of doing this is to give Clomiphene which encourages the pituitary gland to release more stimulating hormones.

CONGENITAL When a condition is passed down from the parents to the child, it is a congenital one.

CORPUS LUTEUM After the primitive egg has left the ovary, the follicle rapidly shrinks to become a clump of bright yellow cells, the corpus luteum, which produce progesterone, a hormone needed for the maintenance of the endometrium in the days immediately after ovulation.

CYSTIC FIBROSIS A condition found in young children where an imperfect secretion of mucus occurs wherever mucus is made. Principal problems resulting are in the lungs, where thick gooey mucus obstructs the air passages, or in the intestinal tract where digestion of food is imperfect and leads to both malnutrition and the passage of bulky, improperly formed stools.

DOWN'S SYNDROME This is a chromosomal problem which causes a baby to be born with a mental deficiency. There is a characteristic facial feature with slanting wide-set eyes. The chromosome problem is usually an extra chromosome on position 21 (Trisomy 21).

ECHOCARDIOGRAPHY The movement of a pulse of fluid can be examined by reflecting ultrasound waves and measuring the speed and form of the wave. This is done in the echocardiography of the heart and the echoes are reconstructed into a composite picture on a computer screen to give a dynamic picture of the working heart rhythm.

ECLAMPSIA When a woman has fits in pregnancy, she is said to have eclampsia. This is associated with raised blood pressure and protein in the urine. It is a serious condition which has been mostly eliminated by good antenatal care.

ELECTROCARDIOGRAPHY Every time the heart contracts, an electrical discharge occurs and these minute pulses of electricity can be measured. They are put together to form visible waves on a screen or paper trace (electrocardiogram) which can be assessed by an expert to examine the function of the heart.

EMBRYO This term is used for the phase of life of a growing unborn child. From the time that the basic body tissues are made (fourteen days) until the organs are fully formed (about ten weeks) the term embryo is used. After this the child is a fetus and before this time he is termed a pre-embryo.

ENDOMETRIUM The lining of the uterus is shed every month in the non-pregnant woman. This tissue is the endometrium and it becomes the recipient of the fertilized egg when pregnancy starts.

ENZYME All body processes can be speeded up by the presence of catalysts which do not take part in the reaction but enhance its progress. In the body these catalysts are enzymes produced by the body glands.

EPIDEMIOLOGY The science of counting events or disease in medicine is called epidemiology. It provides the quality control to population studies and helps assess the value and usefulness of many methods of treatment.

EPIDURAL When a local anaesthetic is injected into the epidural space, it blocks the nerves after they leave the spinal cord. Hence, the areas of the body supplied by the nerves are numbed. In labour a low back epidural abolishes uterine contraction pains.

FALLOPIAN TUBE The oviduct is a tube passing from the area of the ovary down towards the uterus. It is about four inches long in the average woman and conducts the sperm up towards the immature egg (oocyte), and the fertilized egg down towards the uterus.

FETUS Fetus is the term used for the growing unborn child after the time that the organs are fully formed (approximately ten weeks of gestation) until birth.

FOLLICLE The immature egg (oocyte) matures in a small bubble of fluid in the ovary. This is the follicle and it enlarges until finally the egg is obtruded around day fourteen of the menstrual cycle, by which time the follicle is about 2 cm (¾ in) in diameter.

GAMETE Both the immature egg (oocyte) and the sperm are gametes. They are the sexually transmitted carriers of genetic information which in conjunction with each other give rise to a new individual. Each gamete carries half of the chromosomal message, the oocyte bearing those from the mother and the sperm those from the father.

GESTATION This is an old English word meaning the state of carrying the baby in the womb from conception to delivery. Probably its most common use is when we refer to the number of weeks of gestation, which means the duration of pregnancy.

GONADOTROPHINS In the body all functions are controlled by hormones and enzymes. Some of these are messengers, such as the gonadotrophins which control the activity of the gonads (testis and the ovary). Some gonadotrophins come from the pituitary gland and, in pregnancy, others come from the chorionic tissue of the developing embryo.

HAEMOGLOBIN The blood carries oxygen around the body on molecules of haemoglobin. The oxygen is picked up by haemoglobin in the lungs where oxygen concentration is high and released in the tissues where oxygen concentration is lower.

HIV III Human immune deficiency viruses are in several groups. Those causing AIDS are HIV III.

HYPERTENSION As we grow older our blood pressure rises slightly, but in the pregnancy age group it should be in a low range; if it is above that range the woman is said to be hypertensive. This is associated with problems in supply of nutrients to the placental bed and intrauterine growth of the unborn child.

INGUINAL CANALS Two canals pass through the muscular wall of the abdomen at the bottom end. These are called the inguinal canals, and they allow the male gonads to remain outside the body in the scrotum whilst communicating with the inside of the abdomen through these tubes which carry sperm up for storage in the seminal vesicles, the vasa deferentia. In the female the canals also exist, although they are rudimentary and have no function. It is a potential point of weakness in the abdominal wall and occasionally hernias occur down the inguinal canals.

KARYOMETRIC EXAMINATION In order to examine the chromosomes of a developing embryo they have to be cultured in cells and then photographed and assessed microscopically in a karyometric examination.

LESION A lesion refers to damage produced in the body tissues by disease. For example, scarring of small areas of the heart muscle following rheumatic fever are fibrous lesions.

NUCLEUS The nucleus is the central organizing part of the cell. It contains all the genetic material which carries the pattern of life from one generation to another.

OESTROGENS One of the two major female hormones in the body is oestrogen. It is made in the adrenal gland and in the ovary; during pregnancy it is made by the fetus and transfers back into the mother's bloodstream. Oestrogen is essential to the maintenance of pregnancy and to the metabolism of the growing fetus. In the non-pregnant woman it has an effect on much of the connective tissue, keeping the skin supple and reducing brittleness in the bones.

OSMOSIS Water passes easily across a cell membrane by the process of osmosis: it passes from a lower concentration of chemical substances to a higher concentration until the concentration is equal on both sides of the membrane.

OVARIAN STIMULATION The ovaries produce eggs from the primordial oocytes. This is done under hormonal stimulation from the pituitary gland. From this gland come gonadotrophins which stimulate the egg development and production. An artificial method of encouraging egg production is to block the anti-oestrogens with clomiphene from the pituitary gland. It works in an entirely different way from the gonadotrophins but has the same ultimate effect.

OXYTOCIC DRUG Any substance which causes the uterine muscle to contract is an oxytocic. Examples are ergometrine and syntometrine, which cause a single sustained contraction, or oxytocin and pitocin, which result in repeated rhythmic contractions.

PLACENTA The placenta is the exchange station between the fetus and the mother. At the time of birth it is about 25 cm (10 in) in diameter and 2.5 cm (1 in) thick. It is attached to the mother's uterine wall and all exchange of nutrients and oxygen between mother and fetus takes place across it.

PLACENTA PRAEVIA The placenta which links the fetus to the mother is usually sited in the upper part of the uterus. Very occasionally it is sited in the lower part, and then a part may peel off and lead to bleeding. If labour is allowed, a placenta praevia may separate even more producing very heavy bleeding; more commonly a Caesarean section is performed to deliver the baby.

POSTPARTUM After delivery the woman is in the postpartum phase for about six weeks. During this time the body organs return to their normal non-pregnant state and the mother adjusts to her new relationship with the child.

PRIMORDIAL The primitive or older tissues in a body are described as primordial. The primordial eggs or oocytes are the primitive cells which will, under the correct balance of hormones, develop to potential eggs or secondary oocytes. If one of these leaves the ovary and is fertilized by a sperm, it becomes an ovum or egg.

PROGESTERONE One of the two predominant female sex hormones is progesterone, produced by the adrenal glands, the corpus luteum and, in pregnancy, the placental tissues. One of its major functions is to maintain the state of pregnancy once it has started by suppressing uterine contraction.

RADIOISOTOPE Many elements in chemistry exist in a stable state along with several isotopes, elements with the same chemical character but a different total mass from the sum of its atoms. Some are unstable, and may emit radio waves: they are radioactive. This property is useful in labelling certain elements like carbon so as to measure their passage in the body and examine metabolic pathways.

RHESUS NEGATIVE The human race is divided by the presence or absence in the blood of antibodies to the Rhesus factor, a characteristic we have in common with the Rhesus monkey. 85% of us in the United Kingdom are Rhesus positive, 15% are Rhesus negative. It is an important differentiation for a Rhesus positive gene is dominant and could cause problems to the baby of a Rhesus positive man and a Rhesus negative woman.

SICKLE-CELL DISEASE The red cells of the blood which carry haemoglobin are usually rounded. Occasionally however they are deformed by sickle cell disease, in which case their shape is greatly indented until they look like the letter C, and hence like the sickle that cuts corn. This particular condition occurs more frequently amongst those from the West Indies and Africa and can lead to serious conditions in pregnancy. It is one of the diseases that can be screened for in the prepregnancy period.

SPERM The sperm are made by the male in enormous quantities. They are in the semen and after intercourse some travel up through the uterus to reach the far end of the Fallopian tube. Only one can fertilize the egg to create a future baby.

STEROIDS A steroid is a complex chemical hormone produced by the adrenal gland, by the ovaries and by the testis. Examples are oestrogen, progesterone and testosterone.

TRISOMY Chromosomes which provide the inherited plan in every nucleus of the body are arranged in pairs. Occasionally a third chromosome exists at a given position. If such a trisomy occurs on position 21 it leads to Down's Syndrome; a trisomy on position 18 causes Edward's Syndrome.

ULCERATIVE COLITIS The inner lining of the large bowel (colon) sometimes suffers from a widespread batch of ulcers. These heal intermittently, but then occasionally break out again so that the patient has a continual loss of mucus and sometimes blood in the stool. The condition is probably not an infectious one, but is one of the allergy diseases.

ULTRASOUND Sound waves are what allow us to hear in everyday life. However there are some waves that fall below or above the levels which the human ear can pick up, and ultrasound is in the latter category. It is used to reflect off the surface of the fetus inside the body to create an image on a screen. Ultrasound is extensively used in obstetrics for examination of the fetus.

Further Reading

F.W. Crick and James D. Watson, *The Double Helix*, Weidenfeld & Nicolson; Penguin.

Charles Darwin, *Origin of Species*, Dent; Faber & Faber.

Sir S. Davidson, R. Passmore, J.F. Brock and A.S. Truswell, *Human Nutrition and Dietetics*, Churchill Livingstone.

Alan Emery, *The Elements of Medical Genetics*, Churchill Livingstone.

Janet Lanecoop Plaipol, *The Child Welfare Movement* (out of print).

Catherine Lewis, *Good Food Before Birth*, Unwin Paperbacks.

Catherine Lewis, *Growing Up With Good Food*, Unwin Paperbacks.

Bonnie S. Worthington-Roberts, *Nutrition in Pregnancy*, Mosby.

Useful Addresses

Alcoholics Anonymous
General Office for Great Britain   *London Office*
P O Box 1   11 Redcliffe Gardens
Stonebow House   London SW10
York   Tel: 071-352-3001
Tel: 0904-644026

Association for Improvements in the Maternity Services
  (AIMS)
163 Liverpool Road
London N1 0RF

Brook Advisory Centres
Address and phone number in your local telephone directory
under Brook

Child Poverty Action Group
1 Macklin Street
London WC2B 5NH
Tel: 071-405-5942 (2.00–5.30, Mon–Fri)

Citizens Advice Bureaux
Addresses and phone numbers in your local Yellow Pages
under 'Social service and welfare organizations'

The Family Planning Information Service
27–35 Mortimer Street
London W1N 7RJ
Tel: 071-636-7866

Gingerbread (for single parent families)
35 Wellington Street
London WC2E 7BN
Tel: 071-240-0953

Health and Safety Executive
Baynards House
1 Chepstow Place
London W2 4TF
Tel: 071-229-3456

The Maternity Alliance
15 Britannia Street
London WC1X 9JP
Tel: 071-837-1265

The Miscarriage Association
Dolphin Cottage
4 Ashfield Terrace
Thorpe
Wakefield
West Yorkshire
Tel: 0532-828946

National Childbirth Trust
9 Queensborough Terrace
Bayswater
London W2 3TB
Tel: 071-221-3833

Patients' Association
Room 33
18 Charing Cross Road
London WC2H 0HR
Tel: 071-240-0671

Index

Question Slip

If after reading this book you have a question you would like answered, please write it in the box below and send to me with an SAE. I am afraid only questions sent on this form can be dealt with.

QUESTION:

Send to:

Professor G.V.P. Chamberlain
Department of Obstetrics and Gynaecology
St George's Hospital Medical School
London SW17 0RE

Rose Elliot

Your Very Good Health

With an unquenchable zest and energy for life, Rose Elliot radiates good health and vitality, the result, she believes, of sensible and well-balanced eating habits. And when you read through her delicious and tempting recipes it is difficult to believe that all these rich delights are part of a healthy eating plan.

There is an astonishingly large number of people today who feel overweight, under par, who eat through boredom or stress and are generally not getting the most out of life. For many the pressures of everyday living seem to make healthy eating a practical impossibility. In *Your Very Good Health* Rose Elliot considers all the reasons for bad eating habits and demonstrates how very easy and utterly rewarding a healthy diet can be.

Packed with easy-to-prepare, colourful and tasty recipes, *Your Very Good Health* is the essential cookery book for sensible eating that will give you renewed energy for life. It includes an invaluable section on fibre, sugar, fats and cholesterol, additives and salt, with realistic advice on how to limit these potentially unhealthy constituents in your diet.

With Rose Elliot's help you can indeed enjoy very good health – the tasty way.

A Fontana Original

Rose Elliot's Mother and Baby Book

Rose Elliot's Mother and Baby Book is a unique and invaluable guide to raising a baby on a healthy vegetarian diet. Rooted in practical experience and full of tried and tested recipes, it provides all the information you'll need to know about nutrition before conception, during pregnancy and after the birth.

Rose Elliot has long been recognised as Britain's leading expert on vegetarian food. She has a wide following and has received scores of enthusiastic letters from women who have used her *Mother and Baby Book*. Here she explains fully and clearly the nutritional value of all the basic foods and provides you with a comprehensive and well-balanced range of recipes for you and your baby up to the age of two. An experienced mother herself, Rose Elliot also offers a mass of practical advice on every aspect of motherhood and baby care.

Rose Elliot's Mother and Baby Book is a complete, sensible and deeply reassuring handbook for all mothers and mothers-to-be.

'It is a book I wish I had had when a new mother' *Scotsman*

Fontana Paperbacks

Rudolph Schaffer

Mothering

As yesterday's children, today's parents, or tomorrow's parents-to-be, we all have direct experience of mothering. And yet its nature remains mysterious.

Is it an instinct, from which battering and neglect are rare and pathological deviations, or is it a skill which develops 'on the job'?

Recognizing the complexities of the relations between a mother and her child, Rudolph Schaffer is centrally concerned with the question of whether mothering is essentially a matter of physical care, or of attitude, or of stimulation; or whether on the other hand, it is a reciprocal, synchronized activity in which the role of the infant, even of the new-born, is a far from passive one.

In *Mothering*, Rudolph Schaffer brings together the evidence, drawn from many recent studies and research projects, that can lead us not only to a clearer understanding of what is necessary for effective mothering, but to an assessment of the influence of the child's first attachment on his later emotional life, and of the significance or otherwise of the frequently cited 'blood bond' and 'mother instinct'.

Your Growing Child
The Years from Birth to Adolescence

Dr David Fontana

The *book for today's parent*

Parenthood is the most important job most adults undertake in their lives. Bringing up a child – and coping with his or her changing behaviour and needs – involves making all kinds of decisions, from how to deal with a faddy eater to choosing the right sort of school. Whether your child is easygoing or fractious, shy or belligerent, there are always going to be times when you could do with some guidance.

The best tool for good parenting is a real understanding – of your child, and of your response to and relationship with it. Dr Fontana, parent, teacher, child psychologist and family therapist, is more than qualified to help. *Your Growing Child* is the first book to look at all aspects of a child's psychology, and to explain clearly and in detail the reasons behind the various types of child behaviour at every stage, from birth to adolescence. He illustrates not only how you might deal with a wide range of problems you could encounter – like sleeplessness, bedwetting or tantrums, unpopularity at school or sibling jealousy – but also the part you, as a parent, can play in fostering your child's emotional, psychological and educational growth. And, above all, how to *enjoy* being a parent.

Like other books, *Your Growing Child* covers all the practicalities – the daily care of your baby, teething, toilet training and so on – but it is the first to look comprehensively and systematically beyond the merely practical side to what goes on in a child's mind. Informative but not in the least pedantic, it is an illuminating, reassuring and very readable handbook, and one that all parents will wonder how they could do without.

A FONTANA ORIGINAL

Catherine Garvey

Children's Talk

This is a book about what happens to children's language after they learn their first words. It is about how children use language – in talk. Talk can be with adults, with other children, with strangers or with the family. Studying children's talk reveals their growing mastery of social situations and their developing understanding of the world.

Catherine Garvey's delightful and learned book gives a vivid picture of children's minds through the medium of their talk. But it also explains in detail how that talk can be analysed, and just what it reflects about the child's development. She shows the stages by which children overcome different aspects of talk (turn-taking in conversation, or the use of socially appropriate speech), and emphasizes the centrality of talk to children's development and socialization.